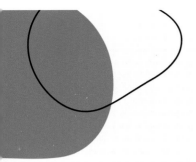

# Copyright

*Thank you*

ⓦ WWW.MONICAFRANKE.
COM

ⓘ clinicontheg
reenmonica

*For all who have come before and all who will come after.*

We are stardust,
crystals,
spirals and curves.
We are powerful
potent,
gentle and ferocious.

We are human.
And we can only be human together.
Let's make it full of
stardust,
crystals,
spirals and curves,
gentle,
potent,
power-with,
ferocious
love.

*Monica*

# Course *Overview*

MONICA FRANKE                    OSTEOPATHY | MIND | MOVEMENT

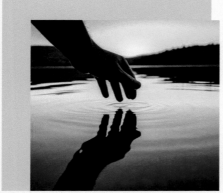

# *Welcome!*
## *This book is designed to support you towards..*

### MOTIVATION & POTENCY

Use the strategies that carry you to your best potential, including recognising and changing course from self sabotage.

### BOUNDARIES & SELF-VALUE

Manage your energy and outcomes by creating boundaries in the relationships which affect your training and progress.

### RELATING FROM WITHIN

Work with an awareness of how mental and emotional processes impact the body

### STRATEGIES FOR SAFETY

Develop understanding and language for how emotional and mental health impacts the body. **Feel Safe, Feel Enough, Meet Your Goals, Build Resilience & Resources**

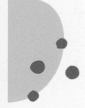

# Meet Monica

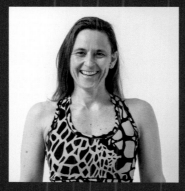

**MONICA FRANKE**
Osteopath | Counsellor |
Movement Expert

---

I have worked in private practice in Oxford and London for 20 years, been a university lecturer, specialised in sports injuries with time spent supporting collegiate athletics, rowing and powerlifting, and then touring internationally with GB Ultimate Frisbee. I love movement, and I am in awe of the human capacity.

I started delving into Transactional Analysis Counselling when I had my teaching job and was having a tough time finding my place. I was also starting to experience that my family structure and my internal world were imploding around this same time. TA in many ways gave me a structural reference to start making sense of this, and over the years I have increasingly used it within my work. The beauty of TA is its accessibility; tools and models that make even complex concepts of counselling and psychotherapy accessible to a wide population.
It is my joy to share this with you.

# *My Why*

This is why I believe BodyBrainHeart is important in fitness and wellness and in building the bridge of change:

Because we need to move to heal. And we need to heal to move.
As I integrate my skills as an osteopath, counsellor and passionate movement advocate, I want to be in a wellness industry that accounts for all of the human. That integrates the understanding, the application and the permission to be more than one thing on any given day and to be able to understand and process all of that - with self-compassion.
When we are the professionals working with people embarking on change, I want to be in a wellness industry that honours the humanity of those people and step into my best self to be with them.

My own fitness journey has been filled with hills and canyons. And as I've travelled those highs and lows, my identity was often aligned with fitness - but in a performative way, rather than a self sustaining and enriched way.
And when the chips were really down, this meant I was lost, low and struggling to find my way out of the dark.

I needed an anchor and a connection.
I needed that connection to believe in me - for who I was right at that worst, hardest moment, and while seeing my potential, didn't feel the need to urge me there.
Didn't want me to perform and show my best self.
Because capacity, beauty and potency are as evident in the moments of struggle as they are in the moments of visible success. In fact, that is the real success.

I truly believe that connecting in a compassionate way with lived experiences, in a way that doesn't need a full disclosure and dissection of details, but in a way that allows this person to be exactly as they are here today. I believe there is such power in that across all walks of life, and no less in fitness. And to let this raise capacity, rather than be dimmed by it.

And so BodyBrainHeart was born. A framework and language that lays the path for you and your clients to pave with your own individual experience, skill, humanness and commitment to both the goal and the relationship, most especially with yourself.

# WHO IS THIS BOOK FOR?

If you have ever reached a point in which you decided you wanted to live in a different way, to experience yourself in a different way, if you wanted to look into the future and see yourself full of vitality, wellness and feeling fit.
Then this is for you.

If your work is with people who have looked into the uncertainty of the future and know they want to be there differently than they are right now, and are willing to make different decisions and do different things to get them there.
Then this is for you.

If you have been in competitive sport and moved to the beat of a particular drum for a long time to stay in it, and now the drum is beating differently.
Then this is for you.

If you understand that change is both exciting and confronting, and are willing to go there anyway.
Then this is for you.

If you want to know how to choose your support team of professionals based on mutuality, belief and curiosity.
Then this is for you.

If you celebrate all the aspects of being human, in a world with other humans and all the beauty the planet offers us.
Then this is for you.

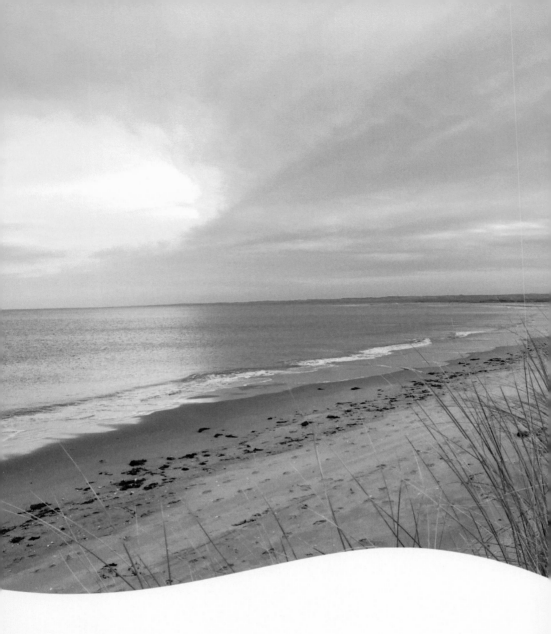

"The secret of change is not in fighting the old, but on building the new."

Socrates

# Pro's – A note about "clients"

Many practitioners of manual medicine will call the people who come in their door "patients". Some call them "guests"and some call them "clients".

Fitness professionals tend to call their people "clients".

So for uniformity and clarity, I have used the term "clients" throughout the book.
Please do take this as whatever terminology you use in your place of work.

# INTRODUCTION

*There is an inner garden inside each one of us, a garden of inner voices.*
*An overly critical inner voice can be brutal to the cultivation of what can flower inside of us.*
*Some of us have been decimated by loss or trauma or tragedy; inside us is a dessert that we believe nothing will grow in again.*
*Whose voice is this? It is even my voice?*
*I have seen again and again -*
*If we begin to give that dessert the vaguest attention, life will come back to life.*

Boyd Varty, 2021
Track Your Life Podcast, Relational Fields

# TRANSACTIONAL ANALYSIS
## What's it all about?

Borne of Eric Berne, MD, (1910-1970) in the late 1950's. Transactional Analysis (TA) is an approach to counselling and psychotherapy certainly - but really to people and the relationships we have. Berne's work focused largely on group therapy, though not to the exclusion of one to one work. From this he developed a style and a theory that is observant, usable and emerges the sediment that often lies underneath human interaction.
Central to this is Parent-Adult-Child model.

## P A C model

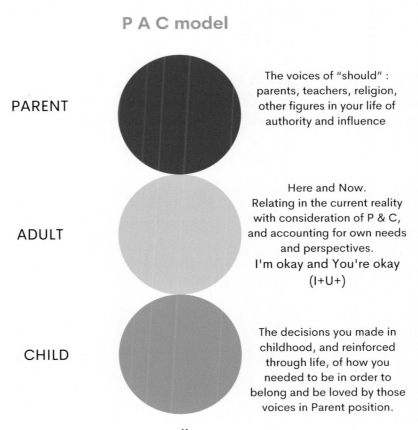

**PARENT**

The voices of "should" : parents, teachers, religion, other figures in your life of authority and influence

**ADULT**

Here and Now.
Relating in the current reality with consideration of P & C, and accounting for own needs and perspectives.
I'm okay and You're okay
(I+U+)

**CHILD**

The decisions you made in childhood, and reinforced through life, of how you needed to be in order to belong and be loved by those voices in Parent position.

I am introducing you in this book, to some of the fundamental concepts of TA and how you can use them, certainly in your relationships with those close to you and with those supporting you towards new intentions. And more than this, supporting you in your relationship with yourself.

**Stress, anxiety, loneliness, trauma**
(UK stats – see next page)
**Effects of covid.**
**The demise of the natural world.**

The modern world – even just the 2020's so far – have challenged our sense of what it means to have a sustained existence on this earth, and then to expand and live a life of wellness, harmony and joy.
So many things are having an impact and it is up to each of us to make new meaning and make new choices.

True to myself, I guess from having lived in so many places around the world, I am most at home when there is a blend and finding ways to integrate. I have embedded my style of working with a variety of modalities.
You will find in this book TA (transactional analysis) theory and How To Use It, Harnessing the Breath, Putting it into Movement practices, science and neuroscience, and embodiment principles.

There is The BodySense Journal as well to accompany you across the bridge.

In my courses, BodyBrainHeart Skills and The Art & Science of Life Changing Coaching, I develop upon the books, with a structured pathway to emerge the sediment and blending further with movement and breathing.

I offer 1-2-1 work as well – whether you are looking for more support on your own personal journey, or if you're a professional looking to support clients in a more integrated way.

I hope you enjoy this book and the journal, and when you need to take it further, I hope you will join me on one of the courses.

# ANXIETY AND LONELINESS IN UK – EARLY MAY 2022

- around 1 in 20 (6%) adults reported feeling lonely always or often in the latest period (5% in the previous period – every two weeks); this increased to around a quarter of adults (25%) who reported feeling lonely always, often or some of the time (23% in the previous period).
- around one in three (34%) adults experienced high levels of anxiety; this proportion was slightly higher among younger adults aged 16 to 29 years (42%) and women (37%).
- Around 9 in 10 (88%) adults reported their cost of living had risen over the past month (91% in the previous period; 13 to 24 April 2022); when we first started asking this question in the period 3 to 14 November 2021, this proportion was 62%.

Office for National Statistics, UK:
https://www.ons.gov.uk/peoplepopulationandcommunity/wellbeing/
bulletins/publicopinionsandsocialtrendsgreatbritain/27aprilto8may2022

# ACCORDING TO UK CHARITY, MIND – APRIL/MAY 2021

Of 12,000 asked, around a third felt their mental health had gotten much worse since March 2020.

https://www.mind.org.uk/coronavirus-we-are-here-for-you/coronavirus-research/

# TRAUMA – UK

- It's estimated that 50-70% of people will experience a trauma at some point in their life. The majority of people exposed to traumatic events experience some short-term distress, but eventually, their trauma fades to a memory – painful, but not destructive.
- Around 20% of people who experience a trauma may go on to develop Post Traumatic Stress Disorder (this equates to 10% of a population). This figure can vary widely between studies, populations and communities researched. For example, the most recent study in the UK, looking at prevalence of PTSD after COVID 19 pandemic, estimated the overall pooled estimate of PTSD prevalence to be 17.52% (double and almost triple than previous estimates).
- 1 in 10 people in the UK are expected to experience PTSD at some point in their lives.

https://www.ptsduk.org/ptsd-stats/

# STRENGTH & VULNERABILITY
## Using The 6 P's

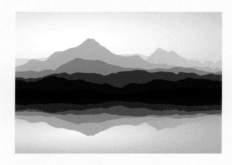

James Clear says, "Every action you take is a vote for the type of person you want to become. True behaviour change is identity change."

When we are looking to resolve a problem and change an aspect of our life, or work with clients who do, we need to be kind to ourself and our stories, and we need a plan.
Whether it's losing weight or losing pain, wanting to be healthier or being able to run 10k, the decisions we have made up to this point, and that lead us to walk into the gym, the running shop or the therapists office, hinge on a set of **perceptions, priorities and predictions**.
Part of our job personally, and the job of all wellness professionals who support us, is to understand that where these have come from are not where we are, and the process of physical change also needs to incorporate a change in these three P's.

And for this I use another 3 P's:
**Protection** - Boundaries, Routines, Your People
**Permission** - I can. I am.
**Potency** - autonomy, mastery-over-time, decision latitude.

When we have these, then our perceptions and predictions about how well things will go become more positive, and it's easier to prioritise our goals and desires with consistency.

*You are not your circumstances. You are your possibilities.*

*Inject Consciousness.*

# CALLING ALL PROFESSIONALS

## *Here & Now*

Below I have posed some questions which are aimed at emerging the values you live by, why they are important to you and how this manifests in your own thoughts and feelings, your body sensations and expressions, and your social self.
And, of course, most importantly here, your professional self.
Being present to yourself paves the way to being present for your clients and supporting them towards their goals.
Here's how to get **Here & Now.**

*I HAVE CREATED 3 PAGES FOR YOU TO WRITE DOWN YOUR THOUGHTS. IT IS REALLY WORTH SPENDING A BIT OF TIME THINKING ABOUT THESE QUESTIONS BEFORE YOU GO ON.*

~ What do you love about your job?
~ Why is it important to you?
~ What do you want for your clients? (eg strong, organised, fun, resilience, choice, etc)
~ What value will it add to give your clients tools that bridge their lived experiences and goals to their inner awareness and capacity?
~ What 3 things bother or upset you when training or treating clients?
~ Have you thought about what's underneath this response in yourself?
~ How does it feel in your body?
~ How do you ask for support or community?
~ With whom do you name your experiences? (incl yourself)

# WORKSHEET

**1**   *What do you love about your job?*

_____

_____

_____

_____

_____

**2**   *Why is it important to you?*

_____

_____

_____

_____

_____

**3**   *What do you want for your clients? (eg strong, organised, fun, resilience, choice, etc)*

_____

_____

_____

_____

_____

# WORKSHEET

**4**   *What value will it add to give your clients tools that bridge their lived experiences and goals to their inner awareness and capacity?*

_____

_____

_____

_____

_____

**5**   *What 3 things bother or upset you when training or treating clients?*

_____

_____

_____

_____

_____

**6**   *Have you thought about what's underneath this response in yourself?*

_____

_____

_____

_____

_____

# WORKSHEET

**7**  *How does it feel in your body?*

_____
_____
_____
_____
_____

**8**  *How do you ask for support or community?*

_____
_____
_____
_____
_____

**9**  *With whom do you name your experiences? (incl yourself)*

_____
_____
_____
_____
_____

# WE ATTRACT OURSELVES
## So Choose Yourself, Too

I think the things that lead a trainer or manual therapist into their profession are the same things that draw particular clients to work with them there.
People inherently recognise when someone can understand and respond to their deep internal experiences of life - even when, and sometimes especially when, they are not even consciously experiencing the emotional impact of that themselves.

To this same end, trainers and therapists demonstrate really effective ways to "rise above", "stay strong", "find their way"...
They often come across as deeply able and sensitively attuned.

And that's not always the whole picture!
Underneath that, there may still be unresolved:
~ uncertainty
~ imposter syndrome
~ body shame
~ conditional regard; that is, valuing themselves based on external and  conditional factors (I'm okay, if...)

And so the feelings of never good enough, exhaustion, spinning your wheels, and the struggle to balance purposeful action with compassion are often all harboured within the internal self of the trainer or therapist.
There is a judder that can be hard to name and integrate.

So, this book is intended to help you navigate your own bridge between surviving and thriving in body, brain and heart. And to offer a framework and language for fitness and wellness professionals and their clients to co-create attuned and boundaried support as you navigate the bridge - making the mental and physical challenges of change an opportunity rather than an obstacle

x

When we are embarking on change, one of the most important elements is the support we seek and building a relationship of trust.

Trust with ourself to make the next right choice for ourselves. It doesn't have to be more than this. You don't have to have it all mapped out. Just make the next right choice towards your vision and intention for yourself and the tomorrow that you want to feel, to live and to be in.

Trust in the people you choose to walk by your side as you navigate your bridge towards change; and lean into the support and strategies on these pages to give you a framework and language that brings grace, agency and inspiration on the days you need it.

Because our relationships are so important - with ourselves and others, especially as we embark on changes and challenges, we're going to explore what being in relationship means, and some of the tools to help you get more clear about how your relationships impact your sense-of-self and your progress.

We're going to talk about:


**RELATIONAL NEEDS**
**ROLES**
**BOUNDARIES**
**TIME STRUCTURE AS A MEANS OF**
**CONNECTING AND DISCONNECTING**
**CONTRACTS**

# Relational beings
# Relational needs

"To be human is to be in relationship with others"

We cannot avoid being connected with others. None of us exists except in relationship; we are born in relationship and need relationships to know who we are in this world. The essence of our humanness is inextricably tied up in our attachments and the ways we relate to others. We are conceived and born within a matrix of relationships and we live all our lives in a world that is inevitably and constantly populated by other humans - even when we are in a fantasy, we are often in relationship with someone, either approaching someone or distancing from someone." (Erskine, Moursund, & Trautmann, 1999).

**Relational needs are the needs unique to interpersonal contact; they are not the basic physiological needs of life, such as food, air or proper temperature. They are the essential psychological elements that enhance the quality of life and the development of a positive sense of self-in-relationship." (Erskine & Trautmann, 1996/97)**

It is a particularly special relationship between a client and a trainer or therapist because as a client we bring extremely personal dimensions of self, and as professionals, being able to offer a space and framework for clients to build their capacity, autonomy and sense of self is hugely important.

**The first way we begin to frame this is by looking at Roles. We then go on to consider Time Structure, Boundaries and Contracts.**

xii

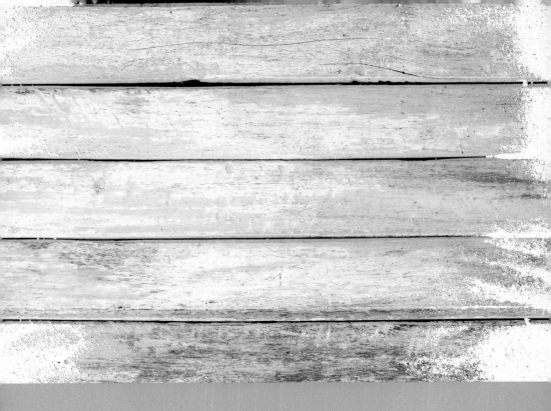

# 1

# ROLES

*You can only inhabit one role at
any given moment.*

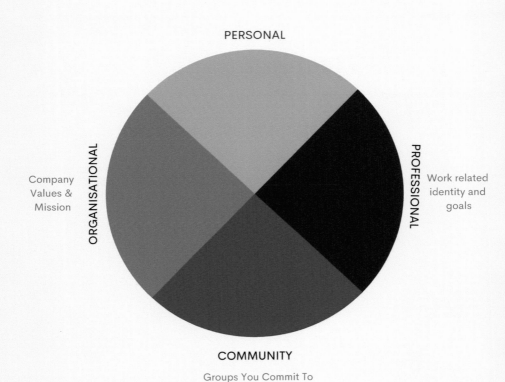

Family, Friendships,
Fitness,
Rest and Reset.
Time for Self.

PERSONAL

ORGANISATIONAL

Company
Values &
Mission

PROFESSIONAL

Work related
identity and
goals

COMMUNITY

Groups You Commit To
& Relate Within

# What features in your role quadrants?

# A WORLD OF
## *ROLES*

*A role is a coherent system of attitudes (T), feelings (F), behaviours (B), perspectives on reality (P), and accompanying relationships (R), which correspond with the environment in which the role is played out in that moment.*

**Bernd Schmid**

When we decide to make a change in our health and fitness, we nearly always look towards the professionals in various wellness fields to get an idea of what we need and how to get it.

We become a 'client' and come to a trainer or health professional in our *personal role*, with very personal needs and vulnerabilities.

The trainer or health professional is in his or her professional role, and will have an organisational role too. This means that being in a social and informal setting has very different implications for each persons' *role experience – their thoughts, feelings, behaviour, perspective on reality and what they need in the relationship.*

During classes and gym participation, there is also an element of community and the culture of the brand or organisation.

Once we know about roles, we can get a better handle on how to manage:

- **Our Own Predictions & Priorities**
- **Goal Setting - What's going to work for us and in what time frame**
- **Boundaries - What's okay and What's not okay - What are your non-negotiables in navigating the bridge towards your intentions.**
- **Contracting - Make it formal - it's not as heavy as it sounds! Let me show you.**
- **Trainer & Therapist Needs - Hey Pros!  We need think about your needs and your boundaries, too.**

We want to create short and long term goals, and it will be important for our support team - the trainer or therapists we choose - to hold the space for us when we are unable to. This might include reminding us that we're always moving forward, framing mid and long term goals, encouraging habit-stacking and anchoring us in the routines and rituals that build confidence and help us to step into our own capacity.

In both settings - training and therapies - it is really helpful to revisit and re-contract for the process intermittently and to consistently use the 6P's to integrate a greater sense-of-self and progress towards health and relationship goals. .

If you are a trainer or therapist, recognise yourself as the containing vessel, the safe space and the guide that holds the framework for the medium and long term plan. You must be resourced and anchored yourself. So going into each session, check in with yourself:

- **In which role quadrant is my energy right now?**
- **What do I need to be 100% in my professional role?**

4

# Roles & Goals

When we are building the bridge towards our wellness goals and we have a co-created relationship with our support team to do that, **we need to mutually commit to:**
**supporting progress, managing expectations, defining short term goals and a process for revisiting long term goals**.
It is useful to get focused on each person's role and needs **in the moment. In this Time & Space you have together.**
Thus, what are your goals as client, and what are the trainer or therapist bringing?

## TRAINING GOAL SETTING

**SHORT TERM**

Client: Motivated & Vulnerable

Trainer brings: Clear Structure, Realistic & Enthusiastic, Invites co-created contract (section 3)

**LONG TERM**

Client: Uncertain of 'If' & 'How '
May become demotivated or disillusioned - needs a clear time structure, mini-contracting and checking in with priorities and permissions.

Trainer brings: Motivation Strategies  (section 7), Boundaries (section 2) & The Four Archetypes (p. 61)

## THERAPY GOAL SETTING

**SHORT TERM**

Client: Uncertain & Vulnerable

Therapist: Allows client to have clear understanding and expectations of problem and journey to resolution, Begins  to update predictions of pain, incapacity and pain avoidance. Sets contract (section 3)

**LONG TERM**

Client: Progress from rehab to increased capacity and pain free living. May see a trainer.

Therapist brings: Moving Towards Allostasis (section 6) Motivation Strategies (section 7) , The Four Archetypes (section 4) & Boundaries (section 2)

May become more dependent

# IF YOU ARE THE TRAINER OR THERAPIST

HOW DO YOU CHECK IN WITH YOURSELF?
AND WHY IS IT IMPORTANT?
IT ENSURES YOU ARE GROUNDED, ACCOUNTING FOR
YOURSELF AND FULLY READY TO SUPPORT YOUR CLIENTS'
SHORT AND LONG TERM GOALS:

- Have you eaten and are you hydrated?
- If you are feeling stressed or anxious, can you take a few minutes of privacy to ground yourself and slow your breathing?
- Are you aware of the next clients goals and ready to work with them?

In order to focus on what that specific person needs in that hour, on the background of their particular goals or health profile, it is so helpful to be fully in your professional role.
It is important to suspend your thoughts, feelings and perspectives of any other any element of your life while you are with a client.

This moment, Here and Now, is **not** about:
- The feelings you have in your personal relationships
- The feelings you have about the organisation you work for
- Your opinions about what the client feels – this would be more about you than them
- Your thoughts, feelings and perspectives of other people in your personal, professional or organisational worlds – this is a road towards false intimacy and loss of boundaries, as well as loss of professionalism.

**STAY IN ROLE
STAY HERE & NOW
STAY CONSISTENT**

**Relational needs** are the component parts of a universal human desire for intimate relationship and secure attachment.

They include:
1) the need for security
2) validation, affirmation, and significance within a relationship
3) acceptance by a stable, dependable, and protective other person
4) the confirmation of personal experience
5) self-definition
6) having an impact on the other person
7) having the other initiate, and
8) expressing love

(Erskine, Moursund & Trautmann, 1999).

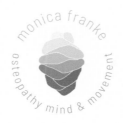

# Relational Needs As Applied To Fitness & Healthcare Settings

When we seek the person or people who will support our journey towards change, we are choosing with whom to form a working relationship that must have a solid base of trust.
And while the relationship is not one of intimacy, it is one of great impact and vulnerability.
Safety in this relational space is so important to really move from one identity to another, one way of living life to another - that includes a healthy, more resilient and self-affirming, compassionate sense-of-self.

I have taken the above relational needs and applied them in the way I see they can underpin the working relationship between trainer or health professional and client.

| Relational Need | Applied in a working space |
|---|---|
| the need for security | to feel a sense of safety and place in the working space; shared values and purpose; mutually accounting contracts |
| validation, affirmation, and significance within a relationship | Receiving positive regard for their commitment and effort; opportunity for decision latitude; they have a part in this co-created journey and that is significant |
| acceptance by a stable, dependable, and protective other person | Professionals who provide autonomy, trustworthiness and appropriate boundaries to the individual and, where relevant, group (classes/ community/ retreats) |
| the confirmation of personal experience | We have unique histories, homes, thoughts and feelings. These can be honoured without needing to know all the details, and as such our agency accounted for with humanity and grace. |
| self-definition | having enough time, space and autonomy to emerge our personal development and identity |
| having an impact on the other person | knowing that what we bring matters to the people we choose |

# Using "Time Structure" To Support Consistency

**"TIME STRUCTURING"** – A way to meet the need for structure when we are with other people. As time is such a big element in service industries, this is a really important lens through which to consider what's going on for us and our clients.

| Time Structure | Contributing To Goals | Diminishing Goals |
| --- | --- | --- |
| WITHDRAWING<br>Lowest relational risk | Doesn't Contribute | Disconnection |
| PASTIMING<br>*chit-chat* | < 10% session | > 10% session |
| RITUALS | Check Prepardeness, Warm Up, Cool Down | Discounting Self-care and Here & Now OKayness |
| ACTIVITY | Meeting Goals | Intensity Too High or Too Low |
| GAMES & RACKETS | Absent in Trainer Guiding Client BackTo Here & Now Goals & Activity | Out of Role Not Holding Boundaries Disregarding Contract |
| INTIMACY<br>Highest relational risk | Celebarting Wins Empathy Appropriate Support | Flirting Relationship Moving Into Personal Feelings & Behaviour |

**WHEN YOU CONSISTENTLY MODEL THE BEHAVIOURS WHICH CONTRIBUTE TO THE GOALS, THE CLIENT IS INVITED TO DO THE SAME. THIS BUILDS TRUST, RESPECT AND RESILIENCE WHEN THE GOING GETS TOUGH.**

*WHAT ELSE is role understanding important for?*

# REFLECTIONS

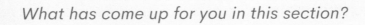

*What has come up for you in this section?*

_____

_____

_____

_____

_____

_____

_____

_____

_____

_____

_____

_____

_____

_____

_____

_____

_____

_____

_____

_____

_____

ROLES                                                    MONICA FRANKE

# 2
# BOUNDARIES

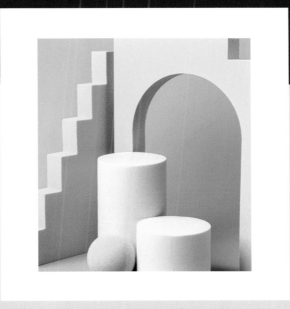

# *Boundaries tell us...*

## WHAT'S OKAY
## &
## WHAT'S NOT OKAY

You know someone has crossed a boundary when you get a
flush of irritation, annoyance - or, let's say it
- **ANGER**!

This is exactly the PURPOSE of anger! It's a good thing and
important information.
It tells us and others what's okay and not okay for us and our
personal time and space.

Many of us don't want or know how to express anger, especially
if doing so wasn't acceptable in our family.
This suppression means two things:
- it gets stuck in our body
- we don't easily sense our own or others' boundaries

So, we may have historic anger that masquerades as something else
(sadness, fear, or even joy)
We may be holding anger in our body - tension, inflammation.
We will feel angry in the moment when our boundaries are not honoured.

Lastly, anger is part of the grief cycle.
And suppressed anger can become depression.
Anger can be the face of fear and shame, showing up as blame.
With anger, there is more often than not a bigger picture.

2. BOUNDARIES                                    MONICA FRANKE

Knowing how to navigate our feelings of anger and frustration is not always easy.
We are relational, we need to initiate contact and know that we have an impact on others. And we need to name boundaries.
This duality can be confusing and hard to navigate with ourselves and others.

And I think it's only fair to say here and now - holding our boundaries, especially across roles - can be lonely.

And we can be lonely and be okay.
It's really worth noticing when we are driving for impact and intimacy in places that are not ours to impact in that way, or that are not going to truly meet our relational needs.

Are we driving with ego?
Are we looking for validation and recognition?

Are we looking in places where we know, when we're really honest, these things are not going to be available to us - not at a deep level that expands our personal or professional experience of the world in a meaningful way.

These experiences leave us feeling confused, empty, rejected, silly and in a negative cycle of "not enough", "I'll never ... xyz."

Know who your people are.
They are the ones you impact, who you can initiate connection with and who will meet you in whatever space you're in and say "You're okay."
You co-create in a meaningful , warming way - that also regulates the nervous system for both of you.
Your people are the ones who will respect your boundaries and who will name their boundaries with you.

## REMEMBER:

Sometimes when we embark on a journey towards change, the biggest challenge is to set our boundaries with those closest to us.

If we can find ways to remove the friction points in our self and our life, then carving out time for fitness and wellbeing can be prioritised enough of the time that we remain resourced. This doesn't always have to look like an hour in the gym - it can be a 20 mins online class or a yoga-meditation flow or three sets of squats and you're done.
Work, kids, spouses and other commitments will benefit when our own resources are nourished and we feel connected to the person we want to be.

# BOUNDARIES WHEN WORKING WITH YOUR SUPPORT TEAM

When we are working with professionals towards our health goals, and especially towards fitness goals, it is really important to remember that difference between the personal and professional roles.
When we are 'the client' we are in our personal role, behaving in social ways whilst feeling both vulnerable and supported by the professional - in their professional role!
You both have a responsibility to hold the boundaries of the relationship. For the professional it's extra important and here's why:

Ethics
Time

# ROLE HIERARCHY
# and BOUNDARIES

A professional has standards to meet. They may be driven by or align with their values, but moreover, they are bound by an ethical framework.
In terms of Roles and Boundaries, we can look at this in two ways.

### Time and Ethics

**TIME** – What was the first relationship (and thus role) that existed?
This is the one that takes precedence.
If it was a therapy (talking or physical, but especially talking) role, this has a very long tail, so it takes precedence even for some time after the therapy has stopped.

**ETHICS** – Talking therapy has the highest ethical standard and thus priority over any other role relationship.
We can consider the hierarchy to be:

Taking therapy
Physical Therapy
Fitness and Movement
Community
Personal

We are going to look a bit more at ethics in the next chapter. I hope this really helps though to think about what's coming up for us in our thoughts, feelings and behaviour. If we're leaning into our trainer or physical therapist alot, there's a chance we're leaning out of our own accountability and the appropriate role boundary.
The same if you're the professional. If you are finding yourself doing this, or finding yourself tolerating this from your clients, have a think about what's behind this for you.
If you find, whatever your role, you're consistently blurring the lines, consider getting some short term talking therapy to explore this and make meaning of it. This is an opportunity for integrating deeper change.

# KNOW AND NAME YOUR EDGES!

By doing this, you are accounting for yourself in the way you would like your people to account for themselves. When we hold our values, vision and boundaries we give others the permission to do the same.

*Your boundaries are valid.*
*And you are allowed to have them in all environments.*
*You can hold both your vision and your boundaries.*

*This allows for more than clairty and respect – it creates bilateral safety.*

Let's say you hate lateness; you can name this in the contracting phase early on in your working relationship with the client. By doing so, you are protecting both yourself and your client by coming to an agreement about the practical arrangements that will work for you both, even in situations of lateness or last minute cancellations.

This means then, that you do not push into the next hour – i.e. your time or your next client's time – because someone else has missed the first seven minutes of their session, even if it was spent in the changing room.
If you did let the client push your time into the next hour, you would be **discounting**:

- your professionalism
- your personal needs and professional boundary
- your right to respect and value of your time and commitent to each client

# BOUNDARIES IN PRACTICE
## Professionals Perspective

**Lateness**

Name the time remaining and what can be done in that time.
Gently confront repeated lateness to establish underlying feelings - avoiding fear of failure, feels embarrassed, struggles with group setting if a group. Are they making enough time around other life commitments to meet their own needs. What else is possible for them to manage time better?

**Fees**

Establish at the outset (contracting) what your fee is and how the client can pay (cash, online, etc). Name your terms (e.g. 7 days) .
If they go through a period when there is less cash available, perhaps agree to do shorter or group sessions for a period. It's often important for clients to know that you can be flexible to changes in their situation without it being either a judgement or an all or nothing. Unless that is what suits you! Then name it!

**Personal Life (Pro's)**

Know what you are comfortable with the client knowing, asking about and commenting on. Sharing our personal information is a journey towards the Intimacy level of Time Structuring (p.10) - this means more vulnerability and more relational risk. We often share things in order to normalise, educate or support a client. If this becomes about comforting them or comforting you - consider other ways in which this can be achieved without sharing this level of personal information.

**Personal Life (Clients)**

It is great to get an understanding of a clients personal situations to the degree that it tells you about their resources.  You, of course, are also one of their resources. Your role is specific and has a specific environmental setting; it should not be used to replace the clients' other resources in their life - either themselves, their relationships or their own thinking.

# BOUNDARIES  IN PRACTICE
## Professionals Perspective

**Time At End**

This can be a really tough one!  The work is done, the time has nearly ended and the client wants to chitter chatter, over-running into the next session or your break.  Hellos and Goodbyes are ritual elements and lower intimacy, in terms of time structuring. The client is essentially trying to maintain higher connection and intimacy.  Strategies  for countering this can include: Naming the time needed for you to re-resource yourself before the next client gets your attention; celebrating something specific about the session that you thought went well; naming a specific focus for the coming week and asking the client to name their strategy for this goal and how they will celebrate. Reiterate your own need for self care space between clients and say goodbye.

**Expectations of Your Role**

Sometimes when clients get frustrated with themselves or the process, they can  - often quite unconsciously - divert that energy onto you. This becomes a narrative about you n being good enough or failing them in the task.  For this reason, I really believe in regular check ins to talk about progress made, the next 1-2 short term goals and how to achieve them, as well as the big long term picture - has it changed, has the path changed? If you're already at the point of tension, approach with compassion - what have yc lost sight of (you're not infallible)? What do they feel, what do they need? Where did the two of you as a team diverge from the path?  This moment is an opportunity to tell the client what they've done well, that you are there with them the struggle, own what you haven't done well, and reaffirm your commitment to them and the process, so that they car do the same.

**Hrs of Business & Availablility**

Last but by no means least!  Be clear from the beginning wl hours you will respond to calls and what hours you will respond to texts. Don't deviate from this!

# Is It Ethical?

We can use the Ethical Grid (next page) as a reference point to consider who is involved and to what end professionals' behaviours and the clients' behaviours (as well as other peripheral relationships) are grounded in ethical principles.

**What do the Ethical Principles look like for trainer/ therapist   (T) & client (C) in some of our Life Situations above:**

| | CLIENT TAKING TIME AT END OF SESSION | | TRAINER SHARING THEIR OWN PERSONAL LIFE | | CLIENT NOT PAYING FULL FEES WHEN PREVIOUSLY AGREED | |
|---|---|---|---|---|---|---|
| | T | C | T | C | T | C |
| RESPECT | X | ✓ | X | X | X | X |
| EMPOWERMENT | X | ✓ | X | X | X | ✓ |
| PROTECTION | X | X | X | X | X | ✓ |
| RESPONSIBILITY | X | X | X | X | X | X |
| COMMITMENT IN REL'SHIP | X | X | X | X | X | X |

# The Ethical Grid

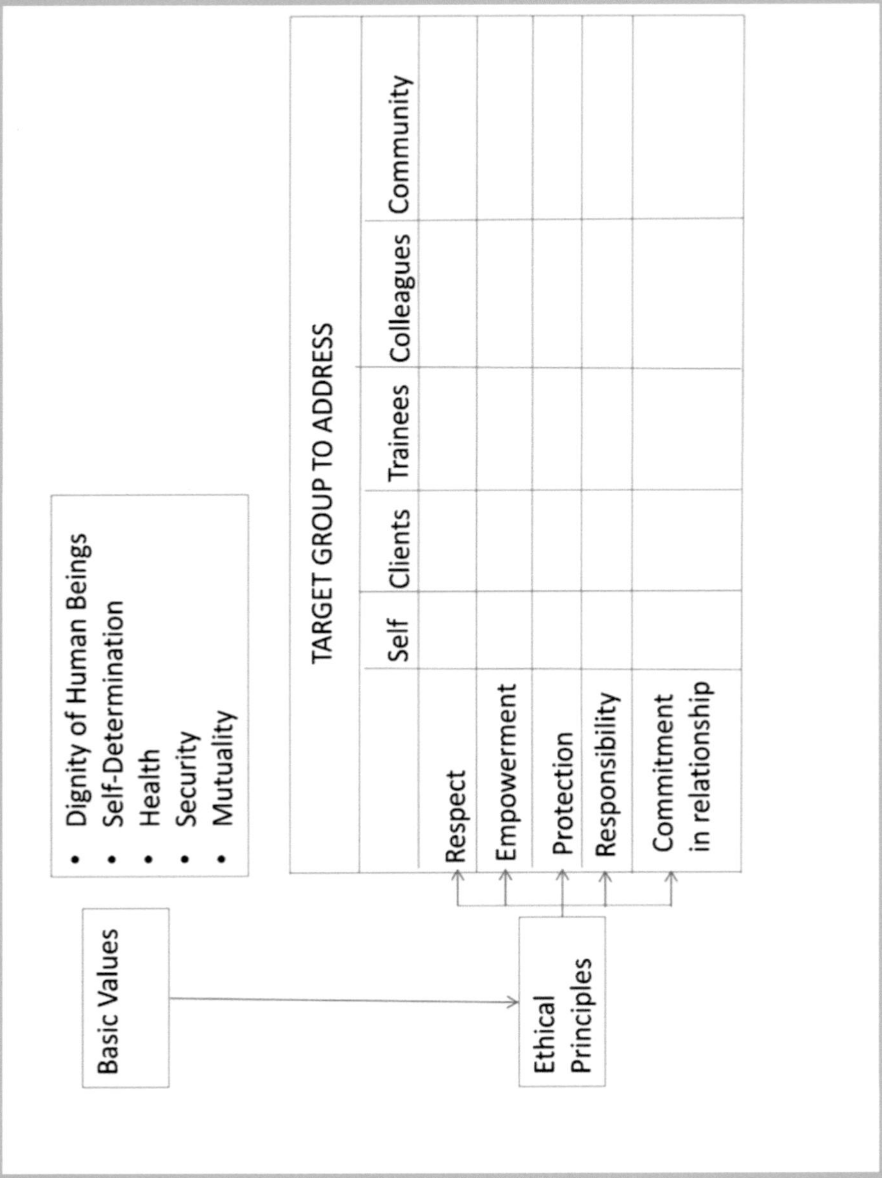
Basic Values
Dignity of Human Beings
Self-Determination
Health
Security
Mutuality
Ethical Principles
TARGET GROUP TO ADDRESS
Self
Clients
Trainees
Colleagues
Community
Respect
Empowerment
Protection
Responsibility
Commitment in relationship

# BOUNDARIES IN PRACTICE
## Client Perspective

**Training Time is Your Time**

When we put a new activity or demand in our schedule, it can impact on our other commitments and relationships. Sometimes this is one of the hardest aspects to navigate in setting about making a change in your life. And the people closest to us, whilst wanting to maintain strong bonds, can be reluctant and nervous about our new direction. Their unconscious fears and feelings of "not enough" can be a real confrontation. You deserve this time and the choice to make a change for yourself. Find way to talk with compassion; and hold your own boundary.

**Trainer is Consistently Late**

Your trainer may have a full list and run sessions close together. Or maybe they don't fully understand the urgency of your time commitment to yourself and your training. If they are consistently late at the start of sessions, it's okay to have that conversation with them to make them more aware of your need to use all of the time for your training session with them.

# BOUNDARIES IN PRACTICE
## Client Perspective

Respecting the trainers time at the end of the session

We've all been there - we've worked hard, achieved things we thought we couldn't, felt uplifted by success and camaraderie - and chatted endlessly! Absolutely celebrate! Absolutely connect and plan for the next session! And remember that your trainer may well have clients following you, or may just need time to themselves.

Personal Space

Offer as much respect and personal space as you would prefer someone you work with to offer you. The trainer is in their professional and organisational, working, roles. It's their job to support and guide you. Unless they specifically invite you into their personal life, and you are 100% comfortable and mutually consenting of this, you can value them for the supportive role they are serving as your trainer. If you do become friends, then training time is still separate to your friendship, and the respect and focus for your goals and how to get there can remain.

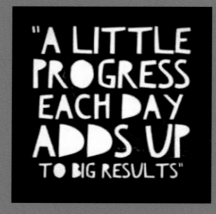

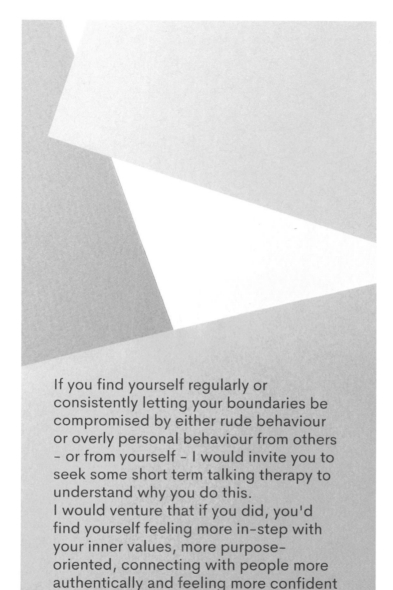

If you find yourself regularly or consistently letting your boundaries be compromised by either rude behaviour or overly personal behaviour from others – or from yourself – I would invite you to seek some short term talking therapy to understand why you do this.

I would venture that if you did, you'd find yourself feeling more in-step with your inner values, more purpose-oriented, connecting with people more authentically and feeling more confident and clear in all your relationships.

# Role Transition Zones

One of the biggest principles I have developed for myself and that I talk about again and again, is connecting with Time and Space. Give yourself time and space; give others time and space. Lean into time and space and see what emerges. It might be a calmer, more connected you.

I have found this imagery below helpful for myself and my clients, when it comes to thinking about space in between the roles we inhabit; making the boundaries and connections we hold within them more easily honoured and accounted for. We become less harried, less caught in role-confusion, and more regulated in our nervous system. This model reminds us to allow time and  space for ourselves in the transition zones.

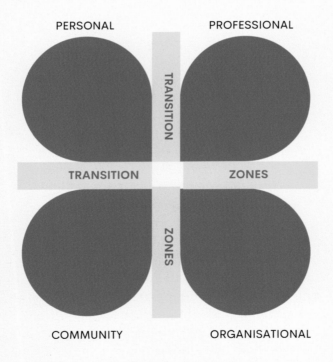

**The Role Butterfly**

# HOW YOU CAN USE THIS

Relational needs are the essential psychological elements that enhance the quality of life and the development of a positive sense of self-in-relationship.

- Recognise Your Need
- Recognise your self as separate from those you are in relationship with
- You can have needs and boundaries at the same time
- You can be separate and together at the same time

- Use the pie chart to identify your roles
- Consider how your needs and values express in different roles
- Get a sense – in your body – of how comfortable each role aligns with your needs and values

"You can only inhabit one role at any given moment."
Depending on our role, and our sense of safety in that role, we will express our values and needs according to what's appropriate and how much vulnerability is possible and permitted, particualrly in group settings.

When you consistently model the behaviours which contribute to the goals and new identity you are moving towards, this increases tolerance, resilience and growth. It also builds trust and teammanship.
We can use Time Structure to indicate how present we are with our goals, with our internal self ,and when and how we might be sabotaging ourselves.

Can you spot where you spend most of your time in the Time Structure chart? How does this help you to NOT achieve your goals?

What unhelpful behaviour would you most like to shed?

# MOVEMENT STRATEGIES TO FURTHER SUPPORT THE PROCESS

- What space are you comfortable with? How do you take up space?

- Spread you arms out to the side, feel as if you pushing an invisible wall. Feel your feet – the whole foot – on the ground. Feel solid and powerful. Breath out fully. What sensations and emotions arise for you here? Whose voice do you hear? Are they helpful and supportive?

- Put both arms out in front of you now. And visualise, feel, this boundary. Who would you like to be inside this boundary? Who do you want to push further back, and who to keep at that distance?

- Soften your arms and knees. Breathe out full breaths, like you're blowing dust off a shelf. Start to swing left and right at your own pace, letting your breath release as you go, let your arms take all the space they need. Go at the pace that feels right and comfortable.

Take a moment to reflect on the roles you occupy, and the space and time you'd like to get that honours your boundaries.

# REFLECTIONS

*What has come up for you in this section?*

_____

_____

_____

_____

_____

_____

_____

_____

_____

_____

_____

_____

_____

_____

_____

_____

_____

_____

_____

_____

# 3. Contracts

*"A contract is a bilateral agreement between 2 or more people."*
*Eric Berne*

A contract is an important and useful way to make explicit the process and practicalities of working towards something with another human, or a group.

Claude Steiner (1974) stated the following as part of four basic requirements of a valid contract, designed for counselling and psychotherapy, but I believe to be relevant for all supported, health oriented goals. They have been used extensively in business, too.
They are:
- mutual consent
- consideration – mutual value
- competency (including ethical diligence), and
- of lawful object (without implying injury to person or property)

Using this as guidance, in addition to the four levels of contracting, minimises the potential for a working relationship to descend into unhelpful or harmful outcomes.

The more that is named and accounted for, the less that can be confused and misconstrued. And in this process, you might discover that the working partnership isn't going to work as well as first thought, and you have a chance to make a different decision.

This can make contracting a confronting process in itself, because we are seeing our own and other people's boundaries, and through this have permission to be fully present in our own needs and motivation. As exciting as that is, it's often new and scary!

A healthy relationship will contract, and also re-contract or mini-contract regularly, as situations and circumstances arise. This forms the basis of ongoing positive communication and trust.

# Levels of Contracting

**01**  ADMINISTRATIVE

**02**  PRACTICAL

**03**  PROFESSIONAL

**04**  PSYCHOLOGICAL

*Contracting is the place in which we can know and name our boundaries*

*It's the first stage to building transparency, mutuality and bilateral trust.*

# The Four Levels

Contractring *in practice*

## Administrative

- Health History Forms
- GDPR
- Confidentiality
- Written contract including practical arrangements

## Practical

- Where
- When
- How long
- Preparedness (consider Maslow's Hierarchy - hydration , nutrition, sleep)
- Boundaries (lateness, cancellations, attire, etc)

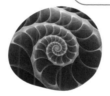

## Professional

- How you use your expertise toward supporting the client to meet their goals
- The process of getting clear on the client's goals and resources
- Leave space for additions as you work together and co-create greater outcomes together.

## Psychological
### EMERGENT

This calls for lots of opportunities to make mini-contracts as you get to know the client, of what is okay and not okay for each of you.

This is where they (and you) hold:
DOUBT   FEAR   GUILT   ANGER
EMBARRESSMENT   SHAME   GRIEF
UNCERTAINTY   TRAUMA
WORRY

# Things to build into the Contract

1. Okayness with discomfort - you can be with it.
2. A structure and strategy for holding space for "sabotage" - give it time and space, and contract for emergent needs at the start. Moments of doubt and uncertainty will arise and you will try to side step them!
3. Sabotage is actually fear - what's going on?
4. Change self-doubt into self-compassion. If we're doubting ourself, we're probably also judging ourself. What needs to be seen, understand, nurtured?
5. Emotional Granularity - tease out the warp and weft of what you're feeling. Use the Feeling Wheel (p.41 ), working from the centre out, and adding your own words as they come up.
6. Emotional Agility - what are the ways that help you move you into a different feeling? Music, journalling, dance and movement are great for shifting your mood. Sound therapy, walking in nature and being with loved ones and pets all work well too.

Resilience is the
capacity to absorb
disturbance to our
frame of reference,
reorganise and create a
new story, a new
identity, which contains
enough of the old to feel
congruent and
recognisably ourselves.

Brain Walker, 2004

# *REFLECTIONS*

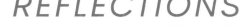

*What has come up for you in this section?*

_____
_____
_____
_____
_____
_____
_____
_____
_____
_____
_____
_____
_____
_____
_____
_____
_____
_____
_____
_____
_____

# 4.

# FROM COMFORT TO GROWTH

*How our connection with ourself will move us to safety, adaptation and growing capacity.*

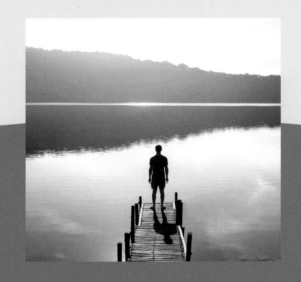

> *It's what we do today that makes our tomorrow*

Practical, Relational & Internal
Processes that Support
Resilience & Growth

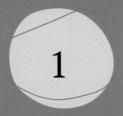

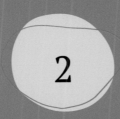

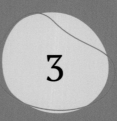

**Routines & Rituals**

**Safety & Trust**

**Intrinsic Motivation**

Develop these practices to pave your way to the life and body you want to live in.
The BodySense Journal is a great tool for you to integrate all of these concepts we're talking about as you begin to make new meaning and the changes that lead to a full and celebratory life.

## Routines & Rituals

These are the repeatable elements of our process that help to anchor us in our capacity and progress. Always checking preparedness, logging sleep and hydration, warming up, reassesseing every 4 weeks. Whatever the elements of your process are, making them our rituals and routines anchors us in that process.

## Safety & Trust

Change is confronting. We need to have people we trust to encourage us, to guide us and to lean into when our own resources are low. It is vulnerable.
We need to feel safe with the people we choose for this role and to be able to work together in mutual trust towards the goal.

## Intrinsic Motivation

One of the key roles of a supportive professional is to helping us find the torch that shines on what is within ourselves . The drive and the will to go through the confrontations of change is there, but oftentimes feels elusive and out of reach. Choosing the right people will catalyse the emergence of these qualities.

# The practice of routine and rituals creates safety

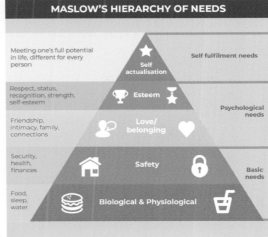

(Models enlarged on next page)

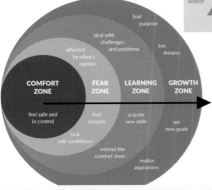

## Safety and trust allows us to move from comfort →growth and self-actualisation

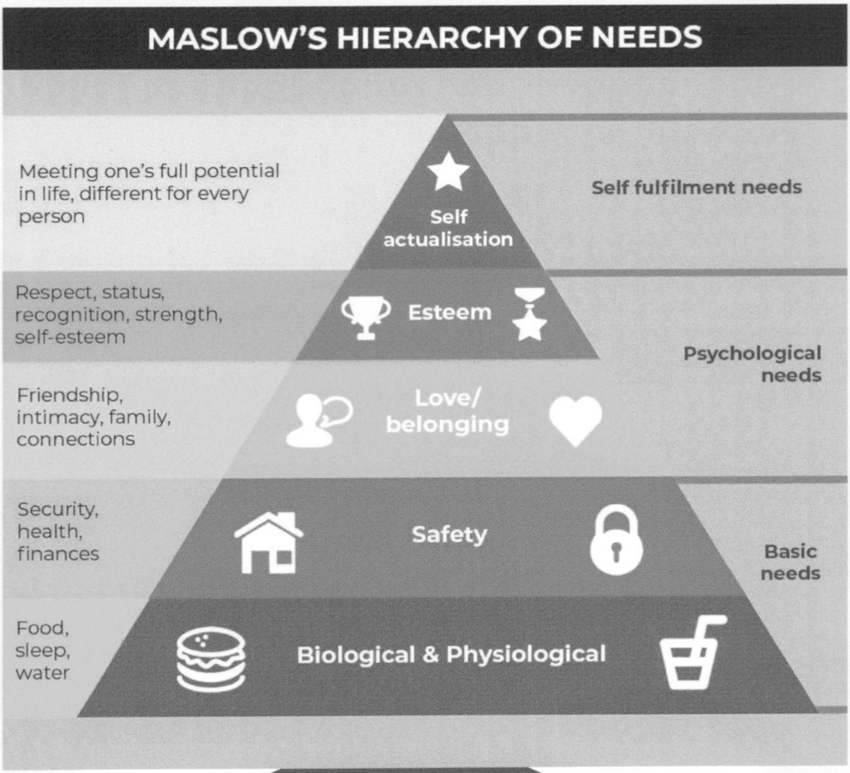
MASLOW'S HIERARCHY OF NEEDS
Meeting one's full potential in life, different for every person
Self actualisation
Self fulfilment needs
Respect, status, recognition, strength, self-esteem
Esteem
Psychological needs
Friendship, intimacy, family, connections
Love/ belonging
Security, health, finances
Safety
Basic needs
Food, sleep, water
Biological & Physiological

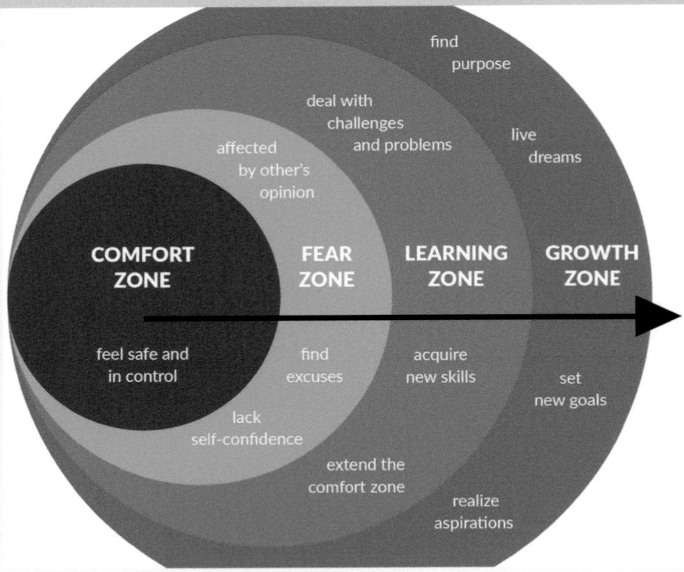
find purpose
deal with challenges and problems
live dreams
affected by other's opinion
COMFORT ZONE
FEAR ZONE
LEARNING ZONE
GROWTH ZONE
feel safe and in control
find excuses
acquire new skills
set new goals
lack self-confidence
extend the comfort zone
realize aspirations

When you're in the learning zone it's a valuable time to name what you are experiencing, and to allow the elements of your new lifestyle habits and identity to be seen.

Every day you make a decision in favour of the direction you're moving in, no matter how small, is a deposit in the bank of being-that-person.

You can be with this even while it's feeling tough or small. Keep your vision; remember the and; trust the bank of you.
That's the difference between fear and learning.

Because –

You will continue to be confronted by such things as:

- moving into new habits and identity might challenge some of the cultural habits you and those around you are used to
- how you feel on the inside no longer matches what you are willing to do to belong in the old role identity and behaviours where your relational needs were not truly met and your habits were discounting your true self
- change is frightening because we are still uncertain of our own capacity and what it will look and feel like to live in this new way
- you may need to set new boundaries for what is okay and what is not okay for you
- you can begin to be more responsible to yourself than to others and the cultures which others create
- You will be met by your own self and others in new ways – you can give yourself permission to have this experience

As we move from old habits, which are comfortable, through fear and learning into growth, we will experience many confronting feelings and choices.

"How do I belong in this space or be this person?
How can I ever be as "x" as that person there?
I am supposed to have it all together - what if I fail?
What if I can't can't handle this?
How will my family and friends react to this new set of values and priorities I'm living by?
How can I assume to make myself important?
Everyone else needs me.."

The pull back to old relational behaviours and the identity that went with them are really hard to confront.

As are the feelings stuffed away in boxes many moons ago-
how to connect
how to be angry
what to do with the grief of loss
what to do with the grief of rejection
the courage to self-define when so many voices and decades want to keep you in a smaller social place
or a different cultural space.

These are all aspects of change.
Of becoming.

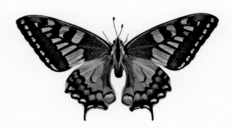

And your trainer or health professional is a privileged witness, advocate and cheerleader of the process.

40

# THE FEELING WHEEL

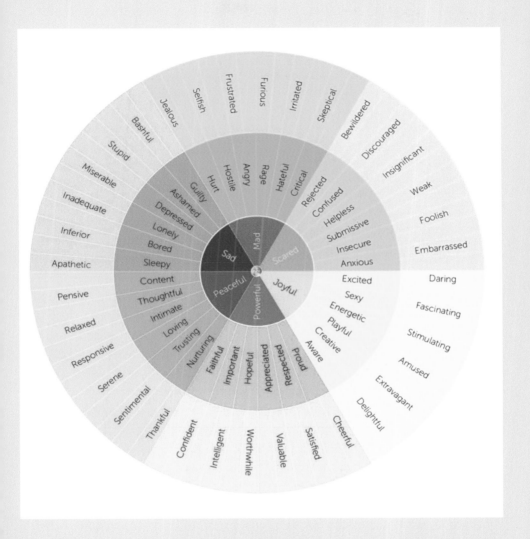

Designed by Gloria Willcox (1982) to help people recognise and
communicate their emotions.
I really like the visual impact of this version and the use of colours to
orient us. This is developed from the work of Plutchick (1980)
connecting emotions and colours.

41

# More About Safety And Expanding Our Health

We will be more able to experience safety when there is nothing calling us to deny, discount or diminish the way in which we experience the world and ourself in the world.

Safety builds in our mind, our body and through our breath. Indeed, our breath is often the bridge between our mind and body, making it a fabulous tool for creating change in many instances.

In transactional analysis, we say that breath is the fastest route to the Here and Now and to Adult (PAC model), p.ii.

## MIND

- Enable The Emotional Landscape – think of your sensations and emotions as a landscape rather than a stake in the ground. This brings perspective and less of a do-or-die feeling. It gives a greater sense of *emotional mobility*. You'll be less likely to get 'stuck' in one emotion if it no longer defines you, even for a short time. When you see it as a landscape, you can visualise moving out of it, and so consciously let go of 'being' one thing and enable yourself to move into and through different emotions.

- Embrace The And – you can experience a number of feelings at the same time. When we embrace this, we reach more broadly into ourselves, it gives us a chance to account for all the feelings. It's possible to be sad and content, angry and compassionate, lonely and at peace.

- Permission To Feel – all the things. There are four core emotions – sadness, anger, fear and joy. (No wonder we humans have negativity bias!) Often, one emotion was "not okay" in our childhood, and so we learnt to mask it with one of the others. Ever felt fear and moved straight to anger? Ever felt sadness and made a joke? There are disowned parts and disowned emotions in all of us. When we start to notice this, give these parts and emotions a little more space and time, we give ourselves permission to feel them, to explore them, to account for them and give them the right shape and size   – not too big, not too small, just right.

- Granularity – get into the weft and warp of what you feel. What's in between, what's beneath, what's twisting on it's side trying to hide?! Do you remember when you were a child and got new colouring pencils – they'd all be organised in descending and ascending shades, blending into each other, creating layers and patterns. This still thrills me! This is how I think of granularity of emotions – the layers, depths, ascending and descending shades. Sometimes they're more like melted wax crayons – explore it all. Take Anger – and now apply the Colouring Pencil Principle. You've got granularity.

- Routines & Rituals – anchor us to ourselves, our goals and our safety

# BODY

We can access safety in the body in a few moments, as well as over a period of time.
There are ways to access and integrate our body systems into long term health, connection and feeling grounded; into trusting and safety in your body.

- **Feet** – Ground yourself. True pronation in the feet is a very positive position and brings a message of groundedness and calm to the nervous system relatively quickly. In movement, this is heightened when we can find our way in and out of the position through the whole leg, pelvis and ribs – and then breathe there. Really own the position and your ability to be there. I incorporate this alot in all of my work now having learnt how to do it well with Postural Restoration Institute (PRI). - with osteopathy clients, movement and always in counselling, we need to get our feet on the ground.
- **Tremoring** – activated by a neurogenic reflex active through the psoas muscle. It is very similar to when animals shake and tremble after a chase, releasing stress after the stressful event has passed. We don't naturally do this as humans, and so it's a positive way to process unprocessed fight and flight reactions and return ourselves back to safety in our neurophysiology. See Tension & Trauma Release Exercises (TRE) by David Berceli - he has a book and a good YouTube video for information and guidance.
- **Gut** – in short, love your gut! Having a healthy digestive system optimises the flow of nutrients as well as optimising your nervous system. There has been an explosion of information on brain-healing nutrition and the gut-brain axis in the last decade, and no bad thing! Take small steps to love your gut every day: eat more slowly, drink enough water, get a range of fibre and vegetables. And beyond that, read some of the books on the gut-brain axis and check in with the recommendations for whatever your preferred diet is.
- **Vision / Vestibulo-Occular Reflex (VOR)** – this may seem a little leftfield, but this is a gaze stabilising reflex; it adjusts eye movement and position as we move our head. Given that the one thing that has to remain during movement is that our eyes stay level with the horizon, then our posture being asymetrical, as it is for most of us, it will activate and make one eye work harder to keep us in a straight line.

- (VOR cont.) When this is activated, the message is "work to do" and goes with "stay alert". Z-Health (www.zhealtheducation.com) offers some great articles and exercises for this, so that we can keep all our movements and muscles moving.
- **Cold water dipping**- stimulates the vagus nerve and helps our body to access the parasympathetic state, as well as boosting immune health and reducing inflammation.  1-3 mins is recommended. I encourage you to use cold in an incremental way that is uncomfortable but not intolerable.
- **Nature, Sunlight & Grounding** - increases many positive hormones and the science of grounding shows direct healing on our cells (REFS below). Being in nature heightens the importance of caring for nature and letting nature care for us. This is very close to my heart.
- **Movement**- last but not least!  It doesn't matter if you choose yoga, weights or qigong, daily and variable movement is a massive contributor to full body and mind health. AND - It's not the only contributor - use a mixture of tools and types of movement. Also, if you mostly use movement and exercise as a way to prove or perform, and it disconnects you from yourself, then it's not healthy. Certainly not for your mind, emotions and even your meaningful relationships.

So, **I invite you to** check in with yourself when you are next exercising.

1. WHICH OF YOUR PERSONAL VALUES ARE MET BY EXERCISING? MAYBE IT'S A VALUE OF COMMITMENT - COMMITMENT TO YOUR FAMILY, COMMITMENT TO YOUR VITALITY IN OLD AGE, MAYBE IT'S COMMITMENT TO ACTIVELY CONTRIBUTING TO YOUR COMMUNITY. MAYBE IT'S A VALUE OF FREEDOM - FREEDOM TO EXPLORE ANY PART OF THE WORLD AND IT'S TERRAINS, FREEDOM TO MOVE WELL AND PLAY, FREEDOM TO EXPRESS YOURSELF.
2. WHEN YOU FEEL GOOD - WHERE DO YOU FEEL THIS IN YOUR BODY? WHAT IS THE INTERNAL NARRATIVE  - THE STORY YOU HAVE ABOUT FEELING GOOD?
3. WHEN YOU FEEL TIRED, UNHAPPY, STRUGGLING SOCIALLY OR EMOTIONALLY - WHERE DO YOU FEEL THIS IS IN YOUR BODY? WHAT IS THE STORY YOU HAVE ABOUT FEELING DOWN?

- REF: https://pubmed.ncbi.nlm.nih.gov/36528336/
- https://pubmed.ncbi.nlm.nih.gov/22291721/
- https://pubmed.ncbi.nlm.nih.gov/18047442/

When you exercise, can you notice and account for all three of these things, without the need to "dumb one down"?
Can you see this moment in a landscape of health, of emotions, of possibilities? And all as a normal and positive part in the tapestry of being human?

The other side of movement and mental fitness I want to talk about is when the sensations in your body and the narratives which accompany them stem for old wounds, trauma, burnout or chronic stress. When these are dominant in our mind, heart and nerves, the process of staying engaged with our capacity, with our vitality and with our power is much bigger battle.

This applies when you are an elite athlete (and with so much performative and social expectation on top), a mum returning to fitness after 15 years (who even am I?) , or a businessman with high cholesterol and a diabetes warning from the doctor.
Or maybe you just saw the effects of COVID and decided now is the time.

Go back to the three invitations above and then add one more invitation:

4. DO YOU KNOW AND TRUST YOUR CAPACITY TO MEET A GIVEN PHYSICAL TASK? WHETHER IT'S LIFT 20KG OFF THE GROUND, RUN 3KM, DO A 20 MIN HATHA YOGA FLOW, COMPETE IN HYROX.

To do this, we need a solid connection to 1, 2 and 3 and a pathway to get there.
Nothing is a problem - it's all just information. And we can work with that.
That's where having a great community, or even just one person who celebrates you, holds space for you and who you trust to be in the process  and make a plan with you (like a really good, person-centred personal trainer) makes all the difference. We have an opportunity to move beyond obstacles of the past.

Never forget that our capacity in't stuck - it can grow.

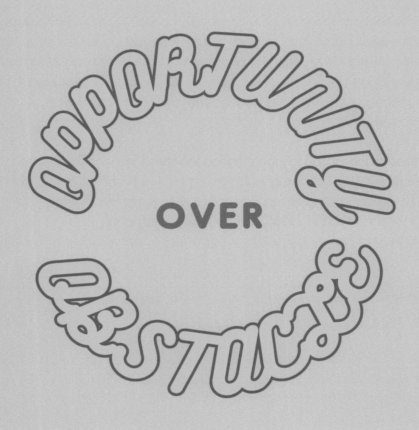

OVER

#OPPORTUNITYOVEROBSTACLE
#BODYBRAINHEART

# BREATH

## THE BREATH IS A BRIDGE BETWEEN BODY & MIND

I am in awe of how powerful the breath is.
It's so everyday.
And yet so deeply connecting and transformative.

A number of books have been written recently about the breath and using it well.
*Breath – James Nestor*
*Oxygen Advantage – Peter McKeown*
*Just Breathe  – Dan Brule*

My experience of intentionally using the breath resides in two main things:

1. **Meditation** – developing the state of inner awareness, letting everything else fall away, just for that moment. Deepak Chopra (honestly, I think a hero of our time) talks about this as being in and expanding the gap that comes after a thought or after a mantra. And, of course, this is deeply restorative. And it allows us to "Listen to the whispers" as Oprah says.
2. **Positional Breathing** – I have already mentioned *Postural Restoration Institute* (PRI) a few times in the book. This is a practice I have worked on myself and with my clients for a few years now. It is also transformative. And accounts not just for the way we move and the ability to build strength on an efficient musculoskeletal system, but also to attend to the nervous system. When we can use both sides of our body in all three planes of motion well – getting into positions and getting out of positions – we can ground, we can jump, we can breathe in with more of our rib and lung capacity and we can breathe out fully. There is constant altering presence of both sympathetic and parasympathetic – both are available. And surely this is an expression of flow (Mihalyi Csikszentmihalyi).

Our breath is the bridge into the present moment, into deeper awareness and connection with ourself and our inner resources. It is the bridge to being fully present Here and Now. From a place of surviving to a place of easy presence and vitality.

# *HOW DO WE USE MOVEMENT TO IMPACT BODY, BRAIN AND HEART ?*

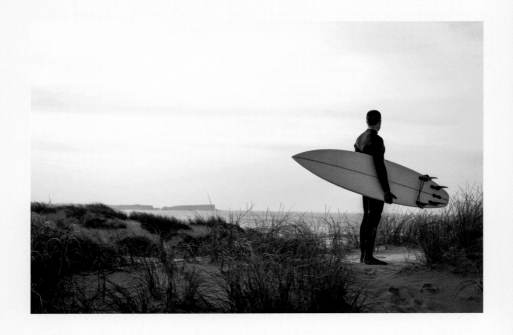

VARIABILITY | POWER | BREATH | INTENTIONALITY

COMMUNITY | SAFETY | INTEGRATION

# WHERE DOES MENTAL AND EMOTIONAL HEALTH FIT WITH FITNESS?

Movement is supposed to be the biggest thing that helps us improve our emotional and mental health, isn't it?! So why not just stop there - why do we need to talk about it?

## THERE IS NO ONE THING

We do not exist in a single state.
We need excitement and we need calm.
We need company and we need solitude.
We need to connect with others and we need to nurture our selves.
We need comfort and we need challenge - even adversity!

Nearly all of the research and all of the books expounding human development and rising to know, meet and remake our capacity talks about all of these things. Yet, when it comes to fitness, it can quickly become performative, aesthetic or proof-of-survival.
It becomes the thing we *Do,* with anything we *Feel* to be taken care of in another box - another time and space.
Or we get stuck in feeling all the confronting, difficult things that keep us in "not enough", "not good enough", "not my place". There is nothing like movement to begin to shake these untruths.

It is so important to continue to integrate *all* the aspects of our self through our movement practices, so that we can know and grow our internal as well as our external capacity. Growth becomes exponential.

We do get a surge of feel good hormones when we work out.
We do gain more confidence by doing the things that are hard and learning we can.
We have greater physical and bio-chemical health when we are working out and moving regularly.

And - the rest of who we are doesn't have to stay at the door and get a dedicated meditation or breathwork session to be met and worked with.

## WE CAN INTEGRATE

# CHOOSING THE RIGHT MOVEMENT FOR THIS MOMENT

At different times, we need different things.

Running, cycling, yoga, weights, conditioning, functional movement, dance, qigong, swimming, team sport.

A high intensity workout will focus us, direct our energy and mind into a specific and narrow purpose, and dissipate the effects of cortisol - for a while.
Turning to a HIIT workout every time you feel stressed, though, isn't necessarily going to sustain your being, in body or mind. High intensity sessions have been shown to increase or maintain stress hormone levels.

Sometimes, even when we want the adrenaline hit, what we actually need is down-regulation.
Slow, connected movement and intentional breath.
This connects us to our deepest self, beyond trauma or chronic stress, and into the real reserve of internal strength that makes us each who we are.

And don't be fooled - this isn't the easy, navel-gazing stuff it might sound like. This slow intentional movement will challenge you, yet connect and calm you deeply. This is where we find our truest capacity to thrive - and that will ultimately bring our greatest gifts.

I think this is one of the biggest lessons and advantages in doing positional breathing work and grounding fully through the feet - that by taking time and space, moving intentionally and breathing intentionally, we can begin to find the anchor within ourselves.

In giving your body and your mechanophysiology time and space, you access the type of nerve fibres that thrive on *slow* - the unmyelinated interoceptors (p. 78 and p.118). This is where we begin to sense and regulate our internal and external mileau. We get a 'felt-sense' and begin 'sense making' of that internal-external interface.

When we notice and name, we gain more awareness of how our experiences and the stories of our life talk to our biology.

**TAKE TIME AND SPACE**
**NOTICE**
**NAME**
**MAKE MEANING (sense making)**
**MAKE NEW MEANING (for the Here and Now)**

When we connect our stories to our biology, then we can know and be present to ourselves exponentially more.
And from here, we have the opportunity to truly expand our capacity as we choose.

You can work consciously with your nervous system and build strength at the same time!
The important part is moving in different ways, being intentional with your breath and naming your own story.

Find your:
**VARIABILITY | POWER | BREATH | INTENTIONALITY**
**COMMUNITY | SAFETY | INTEGRATION**

# CHOOSING NATURE

I believe that connecting with the interface of our internal-external mileau through accessing the interoceptive communication of our nervous system resonates with the interface of our cells and our natural world. When we think about the benefits of grounding and all the microscopic biology within us meeting the surface of our natural world our protons meeting Earth's electrons, oceanic ions, photons of light and phonons of sound - the positive effects of that connection are amplified when we take the time and make the space to connect with nature, morning light, healing sound, bodies of water.
This is a healing path, and it's available to all of us.

# *REFLECTIONS*

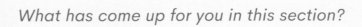

*What has come up for you in this section?*

# WE CAN CONSCIOUSLY BUILD GROWTH & RESILIENCE

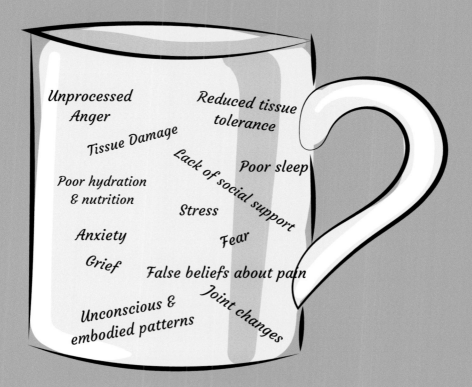

THE CUP ANALOGY as used by Greg Lehman

Our cup overflows when we are unable to
**tolerate or adapt** to the stressors we experience.
It is not about a specific stressor or even number of
stressors, but our ability to tolerate or adapt.

There comes a point where we need to stop just pulling people out of the river. We need to go upstream and find out why they're falling in.

Desmond Tutu

I believe this includes ourselves - at some point, we need to go upstream and find out why we keep falling in.

We should be in constant evolution and adapt to the new without ever losing our essence or our integrity.

Pedro Capo

# USING YOUR MIND, BODY AND BREATH TO INCREASE YOUR STRESS TOLERANCE AND CAPACITY TO PERFORM

- Begin to know your emotions and stressors - name them in your journal. This makes them conscious and begins to account for the effect (and affect) it has on you. It also changes the activity in your brain, moving from the emotion-centred amygdala to action-centred pre-frontal cortex (PFC)
- Notice your sensations - stressors and emotion **can be felt in and influence** - your physiology (e.g. breathing rate, muscle tension, tummy ache)
- -your movement (feeling ungrounded, stiff, favouring a direction of movement and unable to get into the opposite)
- - Your learning - you know some days, things just don't click?! When we are stressed and depleted, also known as allostatic load, one of the things our brain deprioritises first is learning (and movement!)
- This is **all just information**! It's great that our body is talking to us all the time. This information can be used in our journey across the bridge.
- Use it to empower you, and to tolerate and adapt
- This shift can lead to reduced sensations of anxiety, greater confidence and more capacity to learn new things

**NB** - If you have experienced trauma, you may find getting in touch with your inner body sensations triggering. I recommend the excellent and important book by David A. Treleaven *Trauma-Sensitive Mindfulness*. This will help you to recognise unconscious difficulties, when to go slowly in a session and when to seek support from a psychotherapist. Please look after yourself in all your environments.

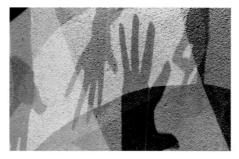

# You Can:

AMPLIFY SLEEP, HYDRATION, NUTRITION

NAME EMOTIONS AND STRESSORS

NOTICE PHYSIOLOGY AND BODY SENSATION

JOURNAL THIS AWARENESS AND IT'S MEANING
TO YOU

GROUND & WALK IN NATURE

TAKE TIME AND SEEK SUPPORT IF IT FEELS
OVERWHELMING

KNOW THAT THIS A WONDERFUL PART OF YOU
AND EMPOWERS YOU TO MOVE TOWARDS YOUR
GOALS

COMMUNICATE IT WITH OTHERS WHEN YOU ARE
IN A SIGNIFICANT PROCESS - YOU WILL BE MORE
TIRED, LESS CO-ORDINATED, LEARN MORE
SLOWLY & REACT MORE STRONGLY TO
TREATMENTS & TRIGGERS - THAT IS OKAY!

TRUST YOURSELF -YOU ARE STILL MOVING
FORWARD

HOLD THE VISION

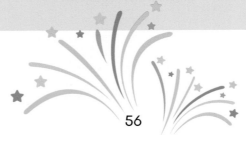

# OTHER TOOLS, DEVELOPED BY ME, TO SUPPORT YOUR JOURNEY

## THE 6 P'S
## and
## THE FOUR ARCHETYPES

These will take all the tools and awareness you've developed so far and let you dive more deeply into your own unique patterns through the lens of established counselling models.

HERE, YOU CAN BEGIN TO INTEGRATE YOUR STORIES
TO STEP INTO YOUR FULL CAPACITY
- IN YOUR BODY, MIND AND RELATIONSHIPS.

## IF YOU WANT TO PUT THIS INTO MOVEMENT

FOLLOW MY YOUTUBE CHANNEL
MONICA FRANKE BODYSENSE AND BREATH
FOR CLASSES THAT COMBINE STRUCTURED MOVEMENT,
SOMATIC FLOWS AND BREATH.

#BODYBRAINHEART

# The 6 P's Model

I first named this "SPIRALS" because of how it felt to me when I had dropped down into this particularly hard, shaming situation and I was naming how to process my way back up through it.
I then realised how integral to my work this processing was, but I wanted a simplified way to explain it. And so, the 6 P's were born!

**You can use The 6 P's as a framework to build your bridge to thriving and celebration. Pave it, decorate it, dance on it  - make it your own!**

Perception  Including your thoughts, feelings and perception on reality, and based largely on previous experiences and environments

Priority  What do you place importance on?
How important do you feel?
How are your needs prioritised amdist all of your roles? Do you priorities align with your goals?

Prediction  Interoceptive- Allostasis (Section 6)
Do you update sufficiently to allow meaningful change based on your current reality?
What support do you need to make updates and new meaning of the sensations they feel.

Protection  What are your boundaries? Can you communicate them explicitly or not?
What is enough activity to help you feel grounded and not overwhelmed? What are your resources for self-care, including training?
This may change forwards or backwards on a given day or month. Allow space for this to emerge.

Permission  I can.
I am.
What do you need to hear, so that you can start saying it to yourself?

Potency  Autonomy, decision latitude, mastery-over-time
Reaching their capacity and potential.
Living a full and celebratory life.

## PERCEPTION
Our brain responds to our perception of reality, not to reality.
Our perceptions develop from the conscious and unconscious narratives based on past experiences and environments

## PRIORITY
How do you prioritise your need for health and healthy activity, compared to all the other things pulling on your time & attention?
How do you prioritise your own values and stay intrinsically motivated?

## PREDICTION
Biologically monitored through "Interoceptive-Allostasis" – interoception is the part of the nervous system which reads and responds.
Allostatic load – is when we our prediction system feels overwhelmed – either by the perception of too much stress, or our perceived  or actual incapacity to tolerate and adapt to it.
Our past experiences, our stories, also lend themselves to prediction going a certain way based on our thoughts and emotions. This is where biography and biology begin to meet.

## PROTECTION
We all need a vessel that will contain us when the ground feels shaky.
This might includetrusted people, your trusted PT, your routines and rituals that anchor you, or your meditation practice. Or all of these!

## PERMISSION
We all need permission – to truly fill our boots
Permission:  To be you, to be important, to think, to feel, to exist, to belong, to be with others,to be separate, to have needs and ask for them to be met.

(TOP TIP:  YOU CAN GIVE YOURSELF PERMISSION ;-)

## POTENCY
Life vitality, capacity, joy, energy, companionship, celebration.
The world needs us, now more than ever, to be our most potent selves

One of the tools we have in the pathway to understanding our own responses to the world around us is what I call The Four Archetypes – four particular ways of feeling (F), thinking (T), behaving (B), perceiving and responding to our environment.

Moving from Comfort to Growth and using different strategies of the Mind, Body and Breath to support us will be in many ways the same for everyone, but each Archetype has something a little different to integrate and different life experiences, which make the particulars of each path unique.
It is what has fed our story (our biography), and been manifest in our perceptions, our biology and body expression.

And it's what can inform our pathway to greater resilience, capacity and joy.

Check out the table on the next page – and if you'd like to download this, I've added a QR code.

My online courses are built to help all the Archetypes develop skills and confidence in building the bridge of The 6 P's through the Body, Brain and Heart.

# THE FOUR ARCHETYPES

I developed these archetypes directly from a piece of TA theory called *Drivers*.

Applied to the process of moving towards greater fitness and health, I highlight the the key strivings, sabotages and needed integrations for four main character types.

I am keen not to overstate these, as it is so easy to put a label on things - and then get stuck in it. To pathologise it in some way.

Our Drivers our fabulous strategies we develop in young childhood to figure out who and what we need to be to get the most love and attention in our environment.

And a bit like inflammation, they are not self-limiting.

We need awareness and an active intervention to make new meaning of who and what we want to be, to be okay *today*.

Let's explore what this might look like for different people.

**PERFECTIONIST**
**PLEASER**
**DISTRACTOR**
**UNSEEN STRONG**

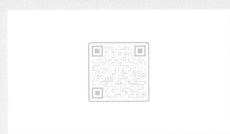

*QR code to Resources page on my website for full Archetypes Overview*

The Archetypes are useful signposts of behaviour and and only one small part of building a picture and a relationship with both our goals and each other.

Outside of this, we can fall inot having a label, which only keeps us stuck.

So the key thing aboutt he Archetypes is that they provide signposts for where the bridge is and how we can begin to cross it.


## PERFECTIONIST

Hits invisible barrier. Fighting themselves.They must get it right. They need to INTEGRATE unconditional acceptance of themselves.


## PLEASER

They must please others but they want to please themselves and to receive instead of just give.

Others come first; their own need and desire is insignificant, they must be "good".

They need to INTEGRATE their value of themselves is above the opinion of others.


## DISTRACTOR

Playful Resistance – they believe if they meet their full potential and success, they will lose relationship.They must keep trying.

They need to INTEGRATE being present to themselves (with feelings and words) in success and know that this is of inherent value from which all potential grows.


## UNSEEN STRONG

Wanting to be connected but needing to stay separate.
I must do it alone, and stand alone. And not necessarily succeed. They must INTEGRATE their own feelings and needs as part of their strength.

"The mind is an embodied and relational process that regulates the flow of energy and information in our body.

DAN SIEGEL

breathe

We're in a time that

"You can no longer leave your humanity
at the door of the workplace."
*Eric Mosley, Work Human*

and

We don't need to leave our humanity at
the door of the gym.

It has never been more important to
integrate our emotions, sensations and
capacity through unconditional
acceptance of our own humanity.
We can be consciously connected
without losing our grit.
We can step into our potency.

When we can meet and care for
ourselves,
we can meet and care for each other;
we can tend and care for the planet.

# *REFLECTIONS*

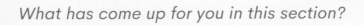

*What has come up for you in this section?*

_____

_____

_____

_____

_____

_____

_____

_____

_____

_____

_____

_____

_____

_____

_____

_____

_____

_____

_____

_____

_____

# 5.

# FROM EMOTIONS TO BODYSENSE

*How we begin to integrate our experiences to feel safe, autonomous and in our full capacity.*

## *Emotions are real.*

"They are events that are an involuntary neurological (a whole body intelligence) response with a beginning, middle and end.

Just about every system in your body responds to the chemical and neurological cascade activated by emotion. Emotion is automatic, instantaneous. It happens everywhere and affects everything."

**Emily & Amelia Nagoski, Burnout.**

This is why safety, trust and practices which move us regularly away from our fight and flight responses are so important. In the context of change, uncertainty and new behaviours, it is helpful to have rituals that we return to for down-regulating our nervous system and being able to oscillate between stress and recovery.

STRATEGIES FOR MOVING THROUGH THE
TUNNELS OF EMOTIONS:
Emily & Amelia Nagoski, Burnout

- PHYSICAL ACTIVITY
- BREATHING
- CONNECTION
- LAUGHTER (& PLAY)
- AFFECTION
- CRYING
- CREATIVE EXPRESSION (& IMAGINATION)

# Exhaustion happens when we get stuck in an emotion.

"Emotions have a beginning, middle and end – to get all the way through the tunnel, we must feel our feelings, and resolve the stress, not just the stressor."

Emily and Amelia Nagoski
Authors of
BURNOUT

We get stuck in our emotions when we don't move all the way through "the tunnel", or don't know how to navigate our way through.
This is especially true of the most difficult emotions:
rage, grief, helplessness, despair and shame.

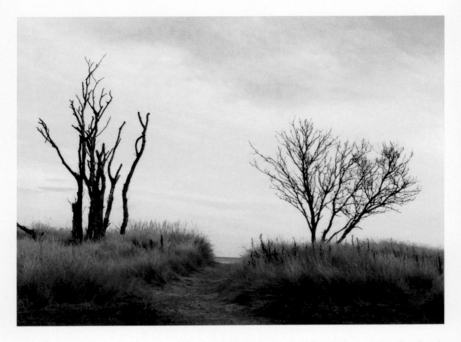

Tentsmuir Beach & Forest, Leuchars, Scotland

As noted by Emily and Amelia Nagoski (Burnout), we must separate the stressor and the stress in order to process our emotions fully, as well as the affect they have in our body systems. We need time and space to recover mentally and physically from stressful events, and to have our resources available for us to have fun, healthy relationships and resilience.

70

We can begin to know our emotions and the emotional affect of situations, and move towards our resources by developing tolerance for the discomfort that affect can bring, as well as strategies that amplify our capacity.

## Developing Tolerance For Discomfort

Sometimes emotions can be quite confrontational, even overwhelming. So one of our resources must be ways of staying in our current reality with trust in ourself.

When the overwhelm is quite acute - we can anchor ourself with visual or auditory anchors that keep us Here and Now. Say the name of those things that are anchoring you, or that you see or hear. For example, name everything in the room of one colour. This process moves us from the amygdala to the pre-frontal cortex.

Feeling our feet on the ground or our back in the chair.

Breathe out slowly to activate the vagus nerve and move out of fight and flight.

When there is not acute overwhelm, but emotion and discomfort are present,  we can use tactile anchors - a stone or trinket that has personal meaning for us, a scarf or fabric we love the feel of. These things can keep us in contact with our grounded self so that we can then move in a way that feels nourishing and supportive, and make contact with our people that are nourishing and supportive.

Notice the affect, name what you feel and the sense you currently make of that in terms of the stories of your life, and then as you stay anchored, make new meaning - recognise your capacity and the bridge you're crossing to the life and self you want to inhabit.

## Amplifying Our Capacity

This is where movement really is a fantastic tool in the box. Movement that feels good, that is varied, and movement that is challenging. Even just 5 minutes of challenging movement and adding strength can remind us what we're capable of, and that includes growth and feeling good. This makes is invaluable.

*Remember*


Sometimes we can be extremely functional – and be anxious and doubtful. Our Drivers, from which the Four Archetypes are derived are strategies we develop in childhood to find our way in the world, be accepted and cope. So, while we may cope very, very well, our nervous system is not necessarily regulated and there isn't necessarily an absence of struggle, anxiety, doubt, fear.

The resources I have spoken of above can help us to recognise and account for the duality of coping and struggling, and give us a pathway to being present to both without feeling overwhelmed or further losing our sense of safety – psychological safety.
We can integrate these aspects of dual experience with compassion and a vision of our true full capacity.

# 6

# EMBODIMENT AND ACCOUNTING FOR INTERNAL PROCESSES

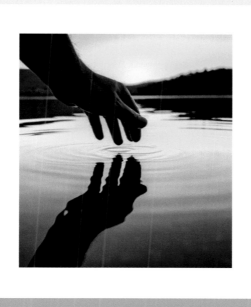

# Who this book is for?

Broadly speaking, if you are human and you have experienced struggles and stuckness in your body, mind or relationships – and you want to be healthy, preferably in all three of these as you grow older, rather than be depleted and dissatisfied – then this book is for you.

More specific to fitness, are you:

- an ex-athlete, trying to regain a sense of self and a new balance to self and life
- a 39 yo mum of 3 who never felt comfortable exercising but wants to start
- a professional athlete experiencing grief or rage mid-season
- a regular sports person, maybe with a family, whose childhood trauma is starting to really surface for the first time and disrupting every feeling, goal and relationship
- the high achieving businessman whose now pre-diabetic and wants to reorder his health and his priorities.

The starting capacity is different, the humanity is not.
The process of struggle is present whether we're fighting up or fighting down.
Pushing physically or being wrung out emotionally.

For some, it's all this at once.
There has to be a process, with routine and ritual.
There have to be human anchors - our people.
We have to have autonomy & decision latitude.
We need to process & update.
We need time & space.
And we must all account for internal processes.

# FTBPR...

*Felling (F), Thinking (T), Behaving (B), Perception (P), Relationship (R)*

Remember right back in Chapter 1, we looked at Roles, as defined by Bernd Schmidt:

*"A role is a coherent system of attitudes (T), feelings (F), behaviours (B), perspectives on reality (P), and accompanying relationships (R), which correspond with the environment in which the role is played out in that moment."*

These are the elements with which we are present and through which we express ourselves in any role at any given moment.
Our F, T, P, B and R are particular to the role we inhabit.

I have added the underpinning unconscious (U) and embodied (E) levels as well, to show what is occurring more continuously "under the radar" so to speak.

This is important to account for, because it's often the unconscious and embodied elements that keeps us stuck in old narratives, in old feelings and old meanings.

AND – We can update!

Updating involves integrating old narratives, the feelings and habits that have held us back and any nervous system dysregulation that's present. We can work with our unconscious and embodied elements to make them conscious and to make new meaning. And working with a counsellor or psychotherapist can make a big difference, especially if there has been long term stress, loss or trauma.

From there, we have more and more awareness and opportunity to keep integrating and accounting for the bridge that exists between our biography – our story – and our biology; and stepping into greater capacity.

| | |
|---|---|
| **F** | *Feelings* |
| **T** | *Thinking* |
| **B** | *Behaviour* |
| **P** | *Perspective* |
| **R** | *Relationship* |
| **U** | *Unconscious* |
| **E** | *Embodied* |

These are the elements with which we are present and through which we express ourselves in any **role** at any given moment.

Our F, T, P, B and R are particular to the role we inhabit. I have added the underpinning unconscious (U) and embodied (E) levels as well, to show what is occurring more continuously "under the radar" so to speak.

## WORKING WITH SUPPORTIVE PROFESSIONALS AS WE CROSS THE BRIDGE OF CHANGE IN HEALTH AND FITNESS

When we start working with professionals who will support our journey and our capacity to change, there is always a psychological element for both people.
Contracting at the psychological level (p.30) is emergent; holding space for it also begins to contract and account for the embodied level of experience.

Checking in and mini-contracting with your support team during or even midway between sessions supports your whole process of change, building your confidence and agency as you update physically and emotionally.

Use your senses and other core organisers (p.112) to check out what's going on within yourself.
You can later reflect on this in your journal, creating a stronger bridge to internal change and resilience.

*The things that are buried in the body are expressed in the body.*

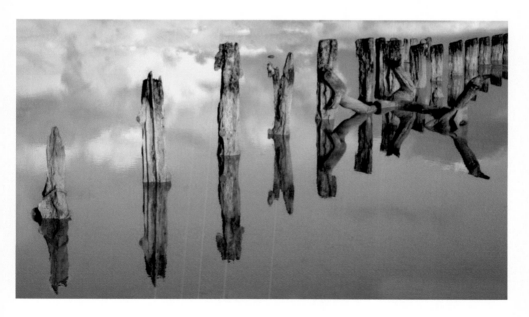

# The Feels

Embodiment comes, in large part, from interoception. This is the neurological pathway which monitors information about our internal and external environments.
These pathways are what we call "unmyelinated"; which means that the messaging is slower and indistinct.

~ Ant (motor and sensorimotor pathways) - fast!
~ Caterpillar (felt experience pathways) - access is best through unfocused, soft attention and given time.

This is why those sensations that arise from our felt-sense are a little indistinct and maybe gauzy. Or like there's static and too much bandwidth for the message being delivered.
They can make us uncomfortable, but these fuzzy feelings, that are difficult to discern where or what, are good!
It's good because that's experiential embodiment at work.

It can be really helpful to get out of your cognitive brain and into your creative brain to interpret and describe these sensations.
What animal would they be?
What colour are they?
What texture, size and shape are they?

My TOP TIP in this process - Don't rush.
This process by it's very nature, needs time and space.
Pause, breath, give yourself permission to be okay with going a little slower, and to feel the feels.

You can be sad and okay.
You can be scared and okay.
You can be relieved and okay.
You can be joyful and okay.

# EMBODIED SELF

Described by Amanda Blake, author of Your Body is Your Brain, as *"the self experiencing itself"*, embodied self-awareness happens through the neural channels we have spoken about, including interoception, proprioception, exteroception and neuroception.

Essentially, it means being able to read the internal and external environments, make emotional meaning of the sensations they bring and choose a response.
Without awareness, our responses will come more from our unconscious - old protective measures that were so valid and wonderful at one time in our life, but haven't been updated, and so the predictions and protections that are generated from this old database might not be helpful now.

Disruptions in our social relationships, and our physical and emotional health may be rooted in these outdated predictive errors, which may be over-protective and not based on current reality.

The unconscious patterns take place via interoception that is unintegrated towards here and now meaning.
We can make new meaning.

**WE CAN UPDATE!**

# BodySense:

How we make meaning and integrate our experiences to feel safe, autonomous and in our full capacity.

It's also really helpful, once you feel your feels, to look underneath them. Sometimes we have another emotion that's been hiding, masquerading as something else.
That is normal, and it's great information.
Remember the Colouring Pencil Principle and Granularity (p. 42) we used to explore the layers and shades of emotions.

We can know our biography and biology much more deeply when we look into these crevices.

Some anger is grief.
Some joy is fear.
Some fear is suppressed excitement.

Look deeper.

*THE EMBODIED KNOWING*
We must have access to our parasympathetic nervous system to reach into this knowing – this is the place of rest, digest and self healing.
This is the pathway to both peace and thriving.

# HOW YOU CAN USE THIS

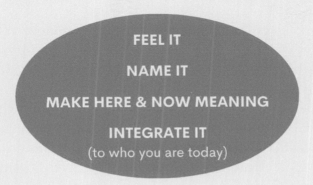

FEEL IT

NAME IT

MAKE HERE & NOW MEANING

INTEGRATE IT
(to who you are today)

So far you have built an understanding of the relationships which exist in different areas of your life, your role in them, and how your values, thinking and feelings arise.
You can understand that different environments and cultures lend themselves to greater or lesser expression, which respectively means deeper or distant connections.
The path to the deeper connections are paved with increased vulnerability and so at some stage there is more risk associated with that - "and even when it feels okay, it is still a leap of faith!"
@brenebrown #vulnerability

You can decide what boundaries you need to have in place in order to take the risk of vulnerability, and to enjoy deeper connections.

When you are connected to yourself first, you can more easily navigate the waters of relationship with others and the confrontation of change in yourself.
You can make new meaning from the experiences you've had and the emotions they bring. And from that, you can integrate them and move yourself more towards the person who does the things you want for your future self.
And you can be more and more of that person every day.

# MOVEMENT & BREATH STRATEGIES TO FURTHER SUPPORT BODYSENSE

- 3 rounds of box breathing followed by two autonomic shift breaths. So BOX: In for a count of 3, hold for 3, out for 3, hold for 3 – repeat three times. Then: breathe in for 4, hold for 2, out for 6, and repeat.
- A yoga flow – Hatha is a great choice here, or tai chi practice
- Turn on the TV! I know – unexpected! Now turn away so that it's to one side of you. Look straight ahead and say "now" every time the image changes. I like to do this to a tennis match or other sport – the pace of change and consistency of environment hit the right mark. This helps to improve peripheral vision and helps our nervous system to feel safe. Do 2 mins on each side – TV on your left and TV on your right.
- Mobilise and massage your feet; do exercises that help you to use the whole range of your foot movement (pronation really isn't a bad thing!) Put a sock under your arch and let your knee glide forward – super slow – and just let the mid foot be heavy on the sock. Take a long, soft breath out. Do a few on each side. Don't rush – really, I can't say that enough.
- Kettlebell and other strength workouts can be great for helping you to feel both grounded and clear in the space and capacity you occupy.
- Building strength is, in itself, capacity building, self affirming and physiologically enhancing. All genders, all ages.
- If you're hypermobile, use lots of bolsters, blocks and bands that give your body extra information about where you are in space. When you put in extra safety in this way, you can let your body work in other ways, including feeling emotional sensations and developing strength work.
- Trauma Release Practice (TRP) – or tremoring – is a great diffuser of nervous tension. Or just shake! Put some beats on and just shake it out! Turning it into a dance is great too!

# FITNESS PROFESSIONALS ..

How do you give TIME & SPACE for a client to think and feel?

When you encourage them to notice and name what their internal experience is, you give them permission to feel the full range of sensations in the moment.

It may feel fluffy to do this – a distraction from the task at hand – but really, you are investing not only in their wellbeing, but also in the depth and breadth of change they are capable of, and in the commitment to a lasting outcome with lots to celebrate.

You don't have to get in the trenches with them, or stop the session to let them go there.
2-3 minutes to notice and mentally put words to what they're experiencing and what it evokes in them is enough.

You can blend this into a conditioning exercise:
"Take a child's pose for one minute – notice what sensations are there.
Put words to it for yourself mentally – maybe you can put this in your journal or training journal later – and then we're going to do some unloaded hip mobility for 2 minutes.
I'm here, I'm watching the time. You don't need to be doing anything different right now. We've got this. You can be with this. Breathe into softly."

And then do another set of deadlifts!
Let them choose – KB's or barbell?

If you do want or need to direct their experience a little more, frame it for them (see Archetypes on p. 61), give a bit more time.
Overall, the process is the same.
And honestly, people can be with it. And move on – connected, happier, more confident.

**"Performance = Actual demands (situation)
+ Expected Demands (our capacity)
*STEVE MAGNESS - DO HARD THINGS.***

"The magic is in aligning the actual and expected demands.
When our assessment of our capabilities (too high or too low) is
out of sync with the demands, we get the schoolchildren version
of performance...
When a mismatch exists, we're more likely to spiral toward
doubts and insecurities, and to ultimately abandon our pursuit."

**Capacity, beauty and potency are
as evident in the moments of
struggle as they are in the
moments of visible success. In
fact, that is the real success.**

In order to perform well, we must be able to assess our own capacity and
stand in that as our reality.
We match the task ahead with our capacity for best performance
outcome.
Our capacity, and knowing our capacity (so many of us under-estimate it),
comes from awareness and connection to our emotional, mental and
physical self. And often through connection with a trusted other person,
like a good personal trainer.

We build our capacity - and our performance - by attending to all of
these.

So let's be with it.
We can be with it.

# FITPRO'S:
## Things that can help a client account for what's going on for themselves internally during a training session..

**01** ✓ "How are you doing?" Make eye contact and let them know you are present to them.

**02** ✓ "Notice just for a moment how this movement / struggle / challenge / progress feels in your body? You can put this in your journal later."

**03** ✓ "What does your emotional self say about that? Is it different from your performing self? It might be helpful to notice this now and reflect on it later in your journal "

**04** ✓ "There's no right or wrong, good or bad. You can be with what's there right now to understand how this experience is for you."

Always reassure clients that the struggle is part of the growth, and being connected to their own thoughts and feelings and making them conscious, especially through writing, allows the opportunity to make new meaning of old messages. And this builds capacity!

## A Fellow Professionals Network..

It is always worth having a list of professionals in your area, or online, that you are confident and connected to.
Having people you can refer your clients to for elements that don't fall into your skill set is invaluable.

And knowing when a client might need some extra support in dealing with the difficult feelings and thoughts that might come up, in order to make new meaning and keep progressing in their work with you, is invaluable too - to them and to you.

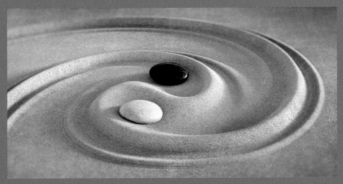

# HOW STRESS AND TRAUMA SHOWS UP AND HOW WE BEGIN TO TALK WITH IT

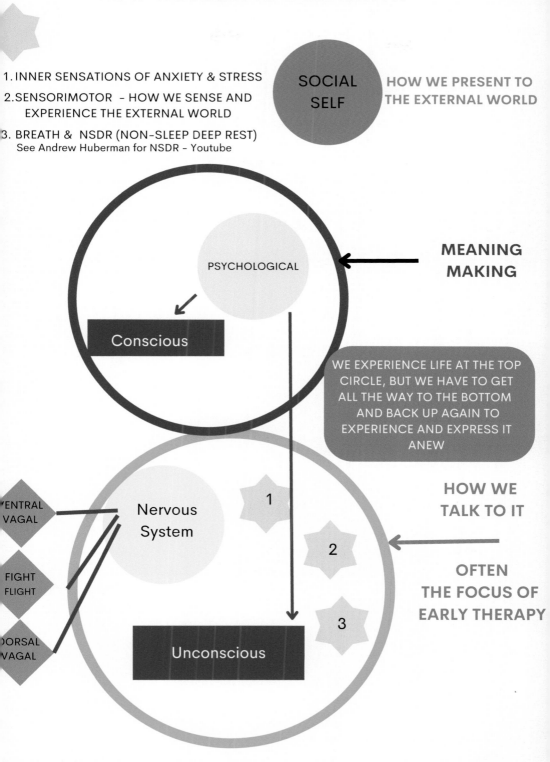

1. INNER SENSATIONS OF ANXIETY & STRESS
2. SENSORIMOTOR - HOW WE SENSE AND EXPERIENCE THE EXTERNAL WORLD
3. BREATH & NSDR (NON-SLEEP DEEP REST)
See Andrew Huberman for NSDR - Youtube

SOCIAL SELF

HOW WE PRESENT TO THE EXTERNAL WORLD

PSYCHOLOGICAL

Conscious

MEANING MAKING

WE EXPERIENCE LIFE AT THE TOP CIRCLE, BUT WE HAVE TO GET ALL THE WAY TO THE BOTTOM AND BACK UP AGAIN TO EXPERIENCE AND EXPRESS IT ANEW

VENTRAL VAGAL

Nervous System

1

FIGHT FLIGHT

2

HOW WE TALK TO IT

DORSAL VAGAL

3

Unconscious

OFTEN THE FOCUS OF EARLY THERAPY

# HOW YOU CAN USE THIS

The unconcious patterns take place via interoception that is unintegrated towards meaning, and so driven by old predictive processing.
We can update!

- Tuning in to our sensations and emotions
- Naming them
- Making meaning of these sensations and emotions in the context of our past, and
- Update the response to the emotions to our current reality
- Integrate them into our experience as we live and set intentions on this day.

- Slow Down.
- Listening to your body as you breathe all the way out.
- Notice and release tension using movement, breath and connection
- Use incremental activation of the CNS to do harder, heavier training - pre-loading, movement patterning & co-contractions help here

Manage loads better to tolerate stress, adapt and thrive

## WE CAN UPDATE!

When we spend some time **connecting to our interoceptive sensations**, and making **here and now meaning,** then it creates a clearer, stronger path towards better relationship with our self and others, and to higher level challenges and training.

Our memories and historic perceptions create an emotional and mental landscape, which we can come to recognise as our embodied self.

# MOVEMENT STRATEGIES TO FURTHER SUPPORT THE PROCESS

- Breathing and yoga flow exercises are great for grounding and regulating; you can take your time, find the movement that is right for your body and go at a pace that feels good on a given day

- Strength workouts are also great for grounding; they help to anchor and regulate the system, and are also very empowering – helping you to find capacities you didn't know you had. I recommend getting a good personal trainer to work with you to support your progress. Remember to use good contracting, boundaries and trustworthy allies

- Use different workout styles depending on your mood and tolerance on a given day; tempo training is great when you feel well resourced and can aid strength gains. On other days, you might choose to focus on mobility and conditioning strategies, including positional breathing. Choose one heavy lift for these days to supplement ongoing progress and the mental and emotional rewards of training outcomes.

- Walks in nature – invaluable for body, mind and nervous system

- Cold water swimming – there has been so much research and chatter about this in recent years, and it's amazing benefit for the vagal system, helping us re-regulate at the centre of our being. Know yourself – if extreme cold is more than uncomfortable, don't go to the usual extremes. 30 secs body only can build resilience and feel invigorating and revitalising.

# *REFLECTIONS*

*What has come up for you in this section?*

# 7

# *ALLOSTASIS &TOLERANCE*

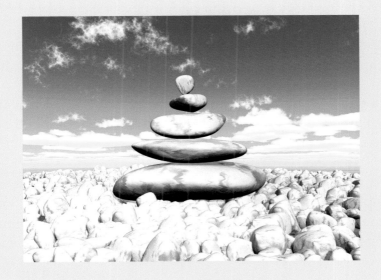

In this section, we look at how
the processes of our body and
mind are interconnected.
The physiology, the
neuroscience, and the inner
meaning.

# Stress, Stressors and Neuroscience

Stress can be physical, mental, emotional or chemical.
We saw from Greg Lehman's Cup Analogy (p.53) that the number or character of stressors in our life is alot less significant than the way in which we tolerate and adapt to stressors.
When we can tolerate and adapt to stress (allostasis), then our nervous system, immune health and capacity for movement is strong.

When our tolerance is overwhelmed, we experience allostatic load and we are more inclined to depletion and disease.
This means that our systemic health, hormone balance and tissue adaptability is compromised. This is where injury and ill health, including the sensations of anxiety, takes place.
We also find new activity takes longer to learn and our nervous system will govern the rate of change we can expect in our tissues.
See pages pages 97 & 98 for more.

We may also be in a situation of compromise from the start, for example, if we have connective tissue disorders like Ehler's Danlos or Hypermobility Disorder – because these conditions make it harder to feel into where the edge of safety is; or where they has been a history of trauma, oppression or depression.

We experience the world, including the loads we tolerate or not, through our feeling, thinking, behaviour, perspective and relating with others, our unconscious and embodied elements.
This is the same **FTBPRUE** we discussed in relation to roles and moving from comfort to growth.

It is largely, of course, through our nervous system - including our brain - that we experience these elements. And the parts that are found to be particularly involved in this are the thalamus, the neocortex and the insula, which modulates the incoming of both external and internal information.

Our internal information is largely communicated through our interoceptors, sensory receptors which detect conscious and unconscious stimuli from our internal environment, including the gut. For this reason, allostasis is often referred to as interoceptive-allostasis.

Allostasis is our prediction system. It's the means by which we read the environment to see if homeostasis will be disrupted and predict what will be needed before homeostatic regulation is called on. When we have errors in prediction  - the reading of information is out of proportion to physical reality - then we are in allostatic load.

One of the other outcomes of allostatic load is sensitisation. This occurs when our system becomes more responsive to the same stimulus, so our tolerance for it becomes lower. Ongoing back pain, for example, can lead to sensitisation because without the right support it is difficult to know what is safe and okay, so we become more cautious and more avoidant.

All of our systems can then become affected by allostatic load; our tissue health and adaptability, our mental health, our hormonal health and how we manage inflammatory conditions caused by the stress response cycle first proposed by Hans Selye.

Seyle proposed that the hormone and chemical cascade (HPA axis) caused by stress, such as cortisol, led to the chronic conditions we know today - diabetes, cardiovascualr disease and autoimmune diseases.

Most illness managed in primary care settings are situations of the stress response cycle (HPA axis) and allostatic load. This includes both our mental tolerance to load and our physiological tolerance to load. The good news is - we can make in-roads to managing these loads better so that we are not depleted and we can tolerate, adapt and thrive.

# HOW?

1. **AWARENESS**- when we start to NOTICE and NAME what we're experiencing, then we're in conversation with our body and our responses. We have conscious control of the impact we're experiencing and the options open to us for response.
2. **MOVEMENT** - movement is nearly always a good option. It improves blood flow, it stimulates movement receptors (proprioceptors) which are happier to move when they experience movement - MOVEMENT BEGETS MOVEMENT 90% of the time. The more you can vary your movement the better -you don't have to be a dancer or a yogi, a pro-athelte or an influencer. Just keep mid range and 4/10 challenging - it's all fabulous information for your body. Movement also stimulates happy hormones - endorphins. And it's often an opportunity to connect with others, if you choose.
3. **BREATHING** - the breath is so powerful that whole books ahve been written about it, movement practices developed around it and it roots us in our very existence!  I'm devoting a chapter on it - Chapter .
4. **COMMUNITY, CREATIVITY, LAUGHTER** - using your senses, playing, moving playfully, engaging in connection and community, laughing - these all heighten wellbeing and remain central to being human.
5. **NATURE** - let nature nourish your sense, your nerves and your heart whenever you can.

The allostatic model, first conceptualized by Sterling and Eyer (1988), emphasizes that organisms do not have to wait until perturbation occurs in order to react; instead, they can rely on learning mechanisms in order to predict disturbances and then proactively act to thwart them.
Allostatic processes can preemptively change the target levels of physiological parameters to maintain the organism's stability in the face of changing environments.

Lisa Feldman Barrett

The discovery of allostasis brought insight to the capacity of the body to be predictive, to learn, instead of just being reactive as in homeostasis.

# INTEROCEPTION, ALLOSTASIS & PREDICTION

There has been increasing research (you can explore some of these from my list of references at the back of the book) in the last decade exploring how the experiences of our external world are filtered, processed and used. This is called 'sense-making' and most information comes in through our senses, and is filtered through the lens of our memory and historic perceptions.

Information also comes into the brain from our body systems – the autonomic visceral and vascular function, neuroendocrine fluctuations and neuroimmune function – this information is known as *interoception*.

The brain constantly monitors *and anticipates* the incoming information from senses and interoception in order to efficiently maintain energy regulation in the body.

*The process of effective prediction from our interoceptive signals is necessary for successful allostasis.*

This is hugely importantly in the arena of health and fitness, as well functioning physiology, pain, decision-making and emotions, as all have a reliance on allostasis and the accuracy of our predictive feedback – of the conversation between our biography and our biology.

When there is an error or breakdown in prediction, like the game Pass It On, allostasis becomes disarrayed and a range of psychological and physiological set backs are experienced.

Allostasis and homeostasis are not mutually exclusive; in fact, they work in concert. The organisation and learning generated by effective allostatic processes allows our systems to be more adaptive and resilient.

" Maintaining allostasis is alot like managing a budget for the body, in which glucose, water, salt and other biological compunds constitute the currency; as with any budget, it's possible to run a metabolic deficit. When this happens, the brain will reduce spending in two "expensive" things: **moving the body and learning new information.** This can result in fatigue, confusion, and anhedonia*, and in the long run, depression."

*Feldman-Barrett, 2019*

*Inability to feel pleasure

Allostatic load is what Feldman-Barrett refers to above as "running a deficit", with reduced coordination and slower rates of learning and embedding new things is the result. I would propose that this lends itself to sensitisation.

This means that the Unconcious and Embodied elements, and the allostatic load which are the result of (and this list is not exhaustive):

Trauma or Childhood ACE;
Collective Trauma (eg War,
Covid, Racism); Burnout;
Post-Natal Depression;
Connective Tissue Disorders

may **need training and movement programs which account for a more gradual progression and also in which great care is made to form consistency, safety and trust.**

# Allostasis & The Processing of Internal and External Stress :
## A FLOW CHART

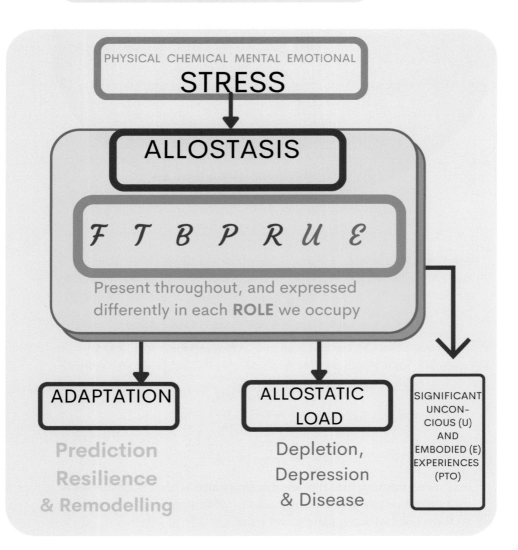

PHYSICAL CHEMICAL MENTAL EMOTIONAL
# STRESS

# ALLOSTASIS

## F T B P R U E

Present throughout, and expressed differently in each **ROLE** we occupy

**ADAPTATION**

Prediction
Resilience
& Remodelling

**ALLOSTATIC LOAD**

Depletion,
Depression
& Disease

SIGNIFICANT UNCON-CIOUS (U) AND EMBODIED (E) EXPERIENCES (PTO)

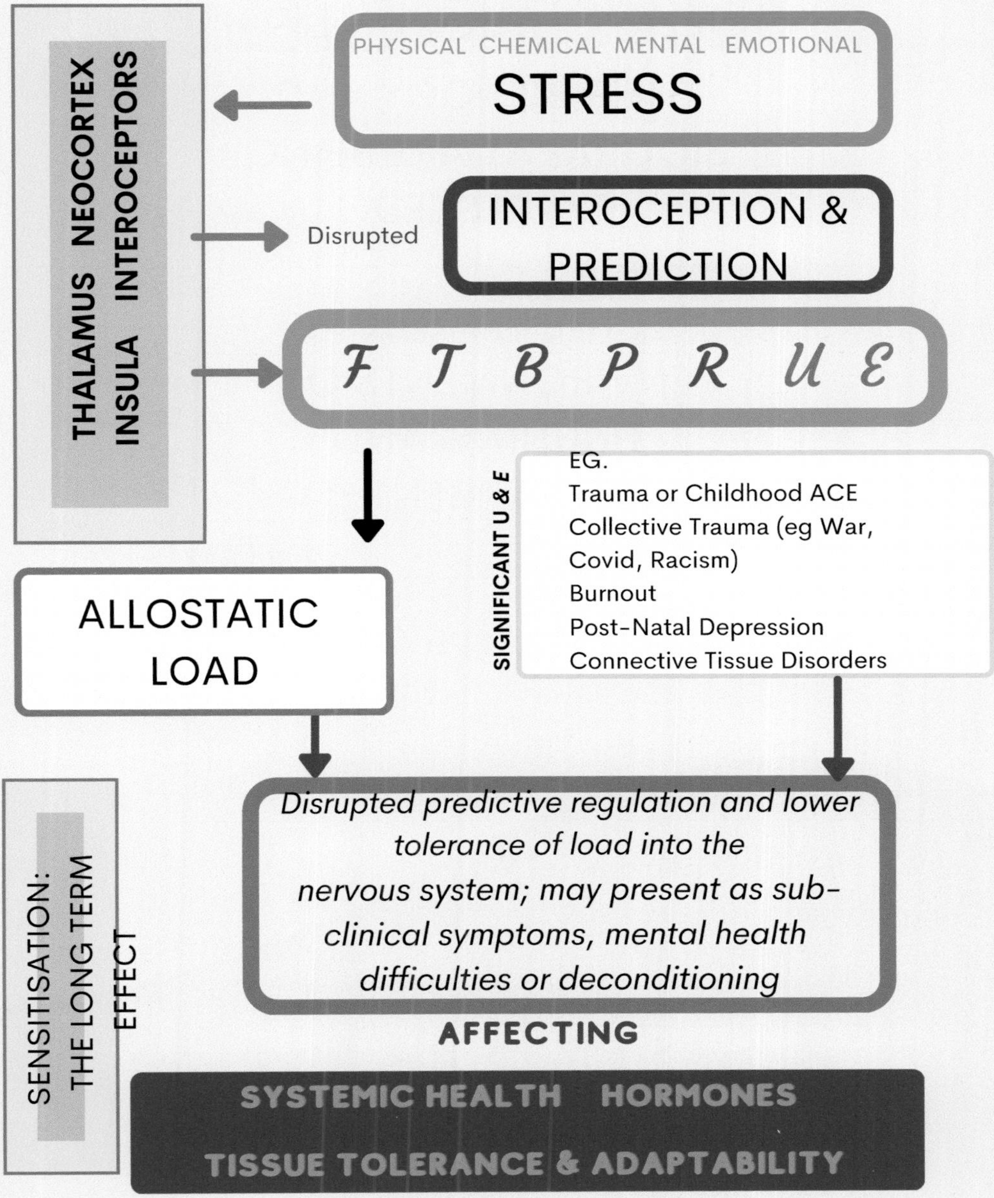
PHYSICAL CHEMICAL MENTAL EMOTIONAL
STRESS
THALAMUS NEOCORTEX
INSULA INTEROCEPTORS
Disrupted
INTEROCEPTION & PREDICTION
F T B P R U E
SIGNIFICANT U & E
EG.
Trauma or Childhood ACE
Collective Trauma (eg War, Covid, Racism)
Burnout
Post-Natal Depression
Connective Tissue Disorders
ALLOSTATIC LOAD
Disrupted predictive regulation and lower tolerance of load into the nervous system; may present as sub-clinical symptoms, mental health difficulties or deconditioning
AFFECTING
SYSTEMIC HEALTH HORMONES
TISSUE TOLERANCE & ADAPTABILITY
SENSITISATION: THE LONG TERM EFFECT

WHAT DOES IT LOOK LIKE
TO ACCOUNT FOR THE
ELEMENTS OF SOMEONE
ELSE'S STRESS AND HOW
THEIR BIOLOGY AND
BIOGRAPHY ARE BEING
EXPRESSED

IN THE PRACTICAL
ENVIRONMENTS OF
TRAINING AND
TREATMENT

LISTEN
NOTICE
NAME
GIVE TIME & SPACE
BE THE VESSEL THAT HOLDS THE SPACE
HOLD NON-JUDGEMENT
KNOW YOUR ROLE
REMEMBER THAT POTENTIAL CAPACITY IS NOT
NECESSARILY THE SAME AS CAPACITY TODAY
(OR THIS WEEK, MONTH OR EVEN YEAR)
& THAT'S OKAY
GIVE THEM DECISION LATITUDE
HELP THEM TO SEE AND STEP INTO TODAYS
CAPACITY
(let them see that feeling emotionally brittle and
honouring that can still mean moving well and being
physically strong)
OPPOSITE ACTION
(a good blast of medball fury can go a long way!)
MAKING A CHANGE IS OKAY
(make it a short session or support them in finding
other ways to resource their BodyBrainHeart today-
nature, creativity, community
CHECK IF THEY NEED OTHER PROFESSIONAL SUPPORT
CELEBRATE THEM

# APPLYING THIS TO TRAINING & REHAB

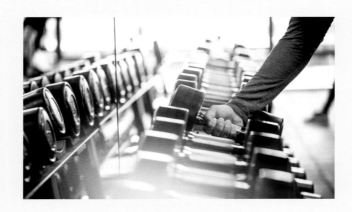

**On days that are more challenging, remember our brain deprioritises two things: movement and learning!  So help them out a bit more in these ways:**

1) **Conditioning & Yoga** – use more references and points of contact, eg bands, blocks and walls to support and align the capacity of the nervous system and tissue adaptability. This is true for hypermobile people too.

2) **Strength** – regress to positions that allow more feedback from the ground. eg if someone is having an anxious day, or is hypermobile and-or menstruating – they still want to train, they still have capacity –AND they need more reference. So instead of deadlifts, for examples, give them weighted bridges for their hinge movement that day.  I also have suggestions for training  strategies and progressions based on The Four Archetypes. **Follow the QR on p. 83.**

3) **Pelvic Floor Health** – allow for lots of time to be able to sense the pelvic floor, relax and integrate it with the breath and grounding contact of the feet. Those who have experienced various forms of physical, emotional and tissue trauma will oftentimes find it very difficult to do this. Indeed, it may be one of the significant limiting factors in their progress in training. A pelvic floor physical therapist can help massively. And remember, it's not only women who have a pelvic floor.

# HEALTHPRO'S:
## Applying this in treatment

**Pain avoidance**
**Sensitisation**
**"My Pain": The Story**

The above are all examples of how clients might be experiencing "predictive pain" and are in or moving towards allostatic load. This is information about the meaning they are making of the sensations of discomfort and reduced mobility – at least in the short term. Unfortunately, they may also make this same meaning in the long term and we can support them by helping them to understand their anatomy and biomechanics, as well as what is generating the sensations.
This gives them an opportunity to update the meaning they make of the impact of sensations on their function, capacity and their life – now and later.

The research shows how sensitisation and fear-avoidance behaviours stem from interoceptive awareness and errors in prediction (see next page).

A significant part of the job as manual therapists and movement coaches is helping clients to understand, update and make new meaning.
This gives people a chance to move out of pain avoidance, stimulate the nervous system in healthy and helpful ways, recover functional movement and comfort, and to tell a new story.

Perception
Priority
Prediction
Protection
Permission
Potency

Consider how you can use the 6 P's in your practice to support clients from their current pain story to their full potential.

102

# Interoceptive Paradigm

## Concepts of Interoception and the "Peripersonal"
## in the Context of Manual Medicine and Fitness

Craig (2013, referenced in D'Alessandro, Cerritelli and Cortelli, 2016) argued that interoception is *"the sensory complement of the autonomic nervous system (ANS), that represents the physiological status of the every tissue in the body."*

Further, *"it is a meta-representation of the perception of self - emerged as a feeling (sentient) entity, which is a pre-stage for emotional awareness."*
(Craig, 2013)
#BODYBRAINHEART

We have seen above that a critical brain centre for interoceptive processes is the insular cortex, which is also implicated in exteroceptive processes, perception of pain, taste, smell and touch.
The insular cortex has been found to be the convergence point of internal and external milieu, producing "body-mapped signals of interoceptive peripersonal space".
(Couto, 2015 referenced by D'Alessandro, Cerritelli and Cortelli, 2016)

If we want to overcome fear-avoidance patterns and to understand our body sensations and update the stories we make about them, we must see that interoception - a big contributor to our sense of self in the world - must be accounted for.

I would also consider the sense of safety, as processed by neuroception (Porges, S. 2009) via the ventral vagus nerve, is relevant in both manual treatment and fitness environments, as the socialising and mobilising expressions of the vagus will be in action.

We will be in contact with these elements of the ourself *and* the people we meet as we move into environments and activities that promote change.

This leads to one of my golden rules:

*Contract For Contact.*

# Contactfulness

Contactfulness doesn't just mean physical contact. Much more than this, it is about how we meet each other as humans relating in our various spheres.

**The unseen elements of interoception and neuroception are at the core of engaging**
**- with others**
**- with ourselves**
**- with new environments and challenges.**

While the expertise and experience are valuable and important parts of the work together, they are secondary to the internal experience of the person showing the will and courage to make a change towards the choice of a healthier, fitter, happier self.

So part of the contract we make is the Contract for Contact – honouring and respecting each other as we meet, agree and commit to crossing the bridge aware of our roles. We can take our time to find our feet (metaphorically and literally), so that we co-create the working relationship, the trust and the bridge to change.

In manual therapies, the emerging research on affective touch can be considered as "interoceptive touch".
**We are contacting - physically and interoceptively - their peripersonal interoceptive field.**
(D'Alessandro, Cerritelli and Cortelli, 2016)

Which leads to my second golden rule:

*Don't Go In Knowing.*

# REFLECTIONS

*What has come up for you in this section?*

# 8.

## INTEGRATING BRAIN AND BEHAVIOUR

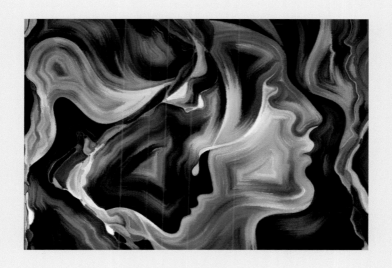

*How we can use our stories, sensations and science to make new meaning.*

# The Psychology & The Science
## - An Overview of Models

**01**

**BIOPSYCHOSOCIAL (BPS)**
Popularised from 2000 onwards as a way to look 'holistically' at an individual. Using the tools in this book, we are taking the BPS model and making it truly relational

**02**

**FTPBR - ROLES & WHAT WE BRING TO THEM**
Originating in Transactional Analysis, these are the ways in which we interact with our environments.

**03**

**5 CORE ORGANISERS**
Coming from sensorimotor psychology, and written about by Pat Ogden among others, the core organisers describe the ways in which we can make contact with ourselves, and from there, express and experience our external environments within a window of tolerance.

**04**

**ONE BRAIN**
From the author and researcher, Feldman-Barrett, this concept reminds us that we have one brain working continuously and as a complex network.

**05**

**MOTIVATION**
Researchers Ryan & Deci (1980) talked extensively about extrinsic and intrinsic motivation. There are many great popular works on this too - Drive by Daniel Pink and 9 Things Successful People Do by Heidi Grant Halverson.

# by Rich Roll @richroll

*Alcohol*
*v.s*
*Running*

"You've just shifted your addiction from alcohol to running."

I hear it all the time.
But here's the thing.

Alcohol is always the easy choice.
Running is always the hard choice.

Alcohol is a way out.
Running is a way in.

Alcohol constricts the mind.
Running expands it.

Alcohol mutes the senses.
Running electrifies perception.

Alcohol removes you from reality.
Running places you squarely in it.

Alcohol fuels false bravado.
Running forces a confrontation with humility.

Alcohol lies.
Running tells the truth.

Alcohol begets denial.
Running begets acceptance.

All roads with alcohol lead to loneliness.
All trails with running lead to community.

Alcohol stole my life.
Running gave birth to a new one.

In other words, alcohol is a prison.
Running is freedom.

Because to drink is to run away.
But to run is to drink in wonder.

 -Rich

We can substitute alcohol for
anything:
food
diets
spending
working
sex

Even exercise, when we use it to
disconnect, as opposed to reconnect.

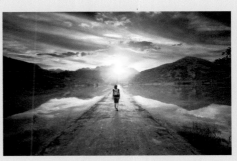

# BIOLOGY TO BIOGRAPHY

### Connecting Allostasis to our
### Roles and Relationships

"The predictions that initiate your actions don't appear out of nowhere... Your brain predicts and prepares your actions based on your past experiences." Lisa Feldman-Barrett.

This particular quote from Lisa Feldman-Barrett, for me, is an explosion of light on **how our biology is connected to our biography** - our story and relationships, our lived experiences and the narratives we draw on the back of them.

Further, the way you feel, think, behave, relate and perceive the world around you is particular to:
- the role you're in in that moment,
- with the constancy of the unconscious, embodied (interoceptive experiences and sense making), and
- predictive processes.

### Meaning Making

It is from our past experiences, our experience of the moment (feeling, thinking, behaving, perspective on reality and relational position) and our current life position - our sense of okayness - from which we make meaning of our place in the world and our interaction with it.

**When we are in our own okayness and we feel good in the world** (I'm ok and you're ok I+U+ #transactionalanalysis ) **then our predictive capacity is less likely to be dysregulated.**

# REMEMBER HOW TO FIND OKAYNESS AND FEEL GOOD IN THE WORLD?

NOTICE
NAME
CONNECT
MAKE NEW MEANING
PRIORITISE
(your self and your health)
SET BOUNDARIES
CHECK YOUR PREDICTIONS
(to meet and grow your capacity)
LEAN INTO YOUR PEOPLE
LAUGH
CREATE
BE IN NATURE
LET NATURE FILL AND HEAL YOU
BREATHE - SLOWLY
MOVE & DANCE
MEET YOUR STRENGTH
(again and again)
NURTURE
(yourself)
FORGIVE
LET GO
GET QUIET
LOVE

# Lisa Feldman-Barrett Quotes
## From her book *Seven and A Half Lessons About The Brain*

### "Brains Make More Than One Kind Of Mind"

"Scientists are still puzzling out how your brain's body-budgeting activities, which are physical, become transformed into affect, which is mental. Hundreds of studies from laboratories around the world, including mine, observe that it happens, yet this transformation from physical signals to mental feelings remains one of the great mysteries of consciousness. It also reaffirms that your body is part of your mind - not in some gauzy, mystical way but in a tangible, biological way."

### "One Brain, Not Three"

"It turns out brains don't become larger over evolutionary time, they reorganise."

"The single region most likely expanded and subdivided to redistribute its responsibilities as our ancestors evolved larger brains and bodies. This arrangement among brain regions - segregating and integrating - creates a more complex brain that can control a larger and more complex body."

Humans "neocortex" is not so much evidence of a triune (triple layered) brain as previously thought, but a brain that reorganises and integrates.

# 5 Core Organisers

## *Building Blocks for Present Experiencing*

**01**   **Cognition**
Thoughts, interpretations of stimuli, meanings, beliefs about ourselves, others, the world

**02**   **Emotion**
The emotions and more subtle nuances of feeling tones mood, "positive" and "negative". See the Feeling Wheel (Gloria Wilcox) p. to explore feelings.

**03**   **Movement Impulses**
Including micromovements and gross motor movement, voluntary and involuntary movement

**04**   **Five Sense Perception**
Inner and outer sensory functions: smell, taste, sight, touch, and hearing

**05**   **Inner Body Sensation**
The physical feeling which is created as the various systems of the body monitor and give feedback about inner states

**According to sensorimotor psychotherapist, Pat Ogden, the way in which someone experiences their body, and expresses and develops body movement is influenced by how they are able to process through their 5 core organisers. The more internal contact someone has, the better that individual is at accessing their sense of self and processing the world around them.
By assessing their reality and trusting their resources, they have greater capacity for accurate prediction and less likelihood for dysregulation and disease.**

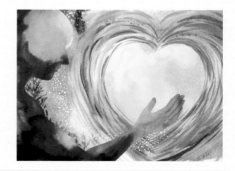

# The 5 Core Organisors,
# The Window of Tolerance &
# Trauma Sensitive Mindfulness

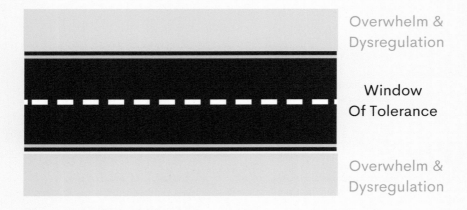

When we begin to experience "not okay" messages within ourselves, either negative self-talk, feeling unsafe our being triggered to some past experience, we move to the edges and sometimes beyond our "Window of Tolerance'.

In this space we become dysregulated – feeling sensations of overwhelm and worry; we experience prediction errors - our internal and behavioural responses may be out of proportion to the reality of the situation; and we may struggle to take in new information or perform challenging tasks.

I liken this to a concept by Jean Ilsley-Clarke ("How Much Is Enough?") talking about parenting - hitting the edge of the WOT is like hitting the dust at the side of the ride. On this terrain, it is easier to get further out of control than get back into control.

Our 5 core organisors are great tools to stay calm and get back on the road.

# *REFLECTIONS*

*What has come up for you in this section?*

# 9.
# MOTIVATION

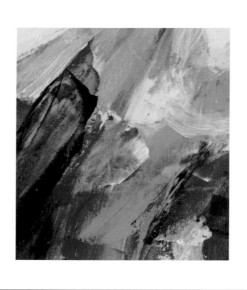

# GOAL DIRECTED ALLOSTASIS

How do we stay motivated when we've reached our goals?!
This is a great reason to intermittently re-contract with your
support team, and with yourself!
Keep Moving. Keep Moving Forward.

- Turn a maintenance goal into a progress goal
- Find Your Why - stay connected to the deeper meaning and motivation for your health
- Seeking greater rewards - reset the goal
- Define your goal with a prevention-oriented focus ("loss aversion") - a great example of this is "I want to take care of myself as best I can as diabetes runs in the family and I want mitigate my likelihood of experiencing that"
- Nurturance & care ("parental type maintenance") - "I want to feel good in my body and have my best energy everyday to do the things I love. I can be healthy."
- Seek autonomy, mastery and purpose (see p. 72) - moving towards good conditioning and strength enhances my capacity and resilience.
- Use If-Then Strategies and Go-To Strategies (see p. 71) use a mixture of these to recognise how far you've come and the person you'd like to continue to be well into the future. Reframing and resetting goals, or finding new ways to express your wellbeing - for example, a dance class, parkour or climbing

### Health Pros

You can support your clients progress by using a mixture of these tools in the
client's management plan.
The treatment aim is always autonomy, function and resilience.
The more we can engender excitement in our clients about these elements
and what that might look like for them, the greater our contribution.

# MORE MOTIVATION

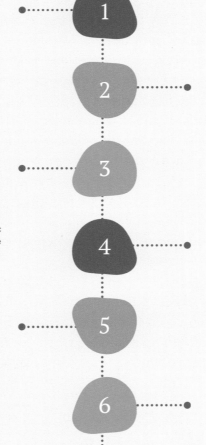

**If–Then Rewards**
p. 54

1

2

**To Date v To Go**
p. 54

**Intrinsic vs Extrinsic Motivation**

A big element of positive psychology, there are some great arguments for intrinsic motivation, starting with the book *Drive*, by Daniel Pink

3

4

**4 T's**

Task, time, technique & team. Defined by Daniel Pink as the elements, which having autonomy over will result in heightened intrinsic motivation

**Decision Latitude**

What are your choices or perceived choices? This is again connected to autonom and thus, intrinsic motivation.

5

6

**Flow**

Defined, in terms of goals and motivation, by researcher Mihalyi Csikszentmihalyi. As described by Daniel Pink, "In flow, goals are clear, feedback is immediate"

**Potency**

# If-Then &
# To-Date vs To-Go
# Thinking

## If-Then
## Thinking

If X happens, then I will do Y."
"If it's Sat at 10am, I will run 3 miles."
"If I want a donut with my coffee, I'll have a glass of water and an apple."

This is a great strategy for short term goals and for catching yourself in a"denying the goals" moment.

Studies show that people who use If–Then Thinking to plan and meet goals were nearly twice as successful at reaching their goals as those who didn't.

## To-Date vs To-Go
## Thinking

"How far I've come"  vs "The distance still to travel."
We tend to naturally use both of these in some conjunction. However, when we get focused more on one than the other, it can produce quite different results.

Predominant "How much further" thinking is useful for spurring you to complete a task you've started. It often heightens motivation and success.

Predominant "How far I've come thinking" can derail us for two reasons: self congratulatory nature hinders or halts further progress; it can also cause us to shift our attention to keep all our tasks bubbling at the same speed, which may mean nothing gets finished!

# X&I
# MOTIVATION

EXTRINSIC

INTRINSIC

Carrots & Sticks

Reward the behaviour sought
and Punish the behaviour
discouraged.

People's motivation is driven
by the external forces acting
on them.

Embedded with:

AUTONOMY
MASTERY
PURPOSE

People can be self
motivated, with myriad
benefits, when these three
elements are facilitated.

## HOW CAN YOU ENHANCE YOUR INTRINSIC MOTIVATION?

- Seek decision latitude as much as possible – KB or barbell today? Strength or Mobility today? Rehab or treatment today?
- Remember the 4 T's for optimising autonomy – Task, Time, Technique, Team
- Connect to your internal process to integrate your sensations, thinking, behaviour and capacity
- Affirm yourself and accept recognition – **humans needs three times** as many expressions of unconditional positive regard as constructive or negative input
- Remember Your Why. What is purpose and how can arrange your priorities to account for this?

MONICA FRANKE

# AUTONOMY
# MASTERY
# PURPOSE

Intrinsic Motivation
Drive
Daniel Pink

*"Flow is becoming one with the music. You find someplace inside the music that you tuck in. And you don't get in the way of the groove. You insert yourself in the song as an instrument. You're no different than the horn, or the snare, or the high hat. It's just smooth and it just flows. I love having that experience."*

Jay-Z
in The Path Made Clear
by Oprah Winfrey

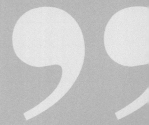

# *REFLECTIONS*

*What has come up for you in this section?*

# What next?
## *Learn how to use these principles more in your work*

If you would like to raise your autonomy, joy and capacity in your own fitness and health, or in working with clients, there are two ways to work with me further.

### ONLINE COURSE

### ONE-TO-ONE SESSIONS

*HARNESSING THE SCIENCE OF REHAB, EMOTIONAL RESILIENCE, NEUROBIOLOGY AND PHYSICAL HEALTH INTO ONE PACKAGE.*
*I CREATE THE BRIDGE FROM THE SURVIVING TO THRIVING.*

### BodySense PROGRAMS

I am delighted to offer a 5 hour webinar-based program BodyBrainHeart Skills, as well as my signature program
The Art & Science of Life Changing Coaching for professionals.

I would love for you to join me!

Please email:
**monica@monicafranke.com**

### BESPOKE 1-2-1

If you would like to work through some specific elements of the workbook as applied to your work, we can do a short series of 1-2-1 sessions online.

I offer an Exploration Session of 30 mins free of charge to identify our fit.

Please email:
**monica@monicafranke.com**

# Thank you so much for joining me in this book!

And for being willing to make 'the work' broader, deeper and more celebratory.

I hope it has stimulated your thoughts and increased your confidence towards making the changes you wish for yourself; how to see and meet the challenges, and how to ask for the expertise, boundaries and connection you need.
I hope the journal, if you have it, serves you well in this process and beyond.

I may not know you, but I am 100% with you, in your challenges and your celebrations.
You Can Do This!

Pros:
Thank you for joining me in this way of supporting the humans who walk through our doors to be their fullest, most potentiated self.

*Monica*

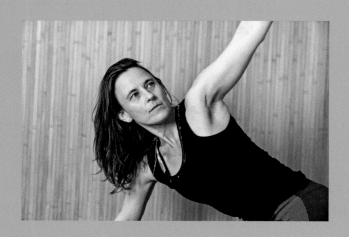

# REFERENCES

1. Achor S. (2018) Big Potential, Virgin,London.
2. Barrett L.F. (2020). Seven and a Half Lessons About The Brain. Picador, London.
3. Barrett L.F., Quigley K.S., Hamilton P. (2016) An active inference of allostasis and interoception in depression Phil. Trans. R. Soc. B 371: 20160011
4. Berne, E. (1974) What Do You Say After You Say Hello? Corgi, London.
5. Berne E. (1964) Games People Play. Penguin Random House, UK.
6. Bernston G.G., Khalsa S.S. (2021) Neural Circuits of INteroception. Trends in Neuroscience 44:1
7. Blake A. (2018) Your Brain is Your Body, Trokay Press.
8. Bienertova-Vasku J., Zlamal F., Necesanek I., Konecny D., Vasku A. (2016) Calcultaimg Stress: From Entopry to a Thermodynamic Concept of Health and Disease. PLoS ONE 11(1):e0146667
9. Bohlen L., Shaw R., Cerritelli F., Esteves J.E. (2021) Osteopathy and Mental Health: An Embodied, Preidctive and Interoceptive Framework. *Frontiers in Psychology*, 10:3389.
10. Cerritelli F. et al, (2020) Effects of mnaul approaches with osteopathic modality on brain correlates of interoception: an fMRI study. *Scientific Reports, Nature Research*, 10:3214
11. Clear J. (2018) Atomic Habits. Penguin Publishing.
12. Corcoran A.W., Hohwy J. (2017) Allostasis, interoception, and the free energy principle: Feeling our way forward. OUP
13. D'Alessandro G., Cerritelli F., Cortelli P. (2016) Sensitization and Interoception as Key Neurlogical Concepts in Ostopathy and Other Manual Medicine. *Frontiers n Neuroscience* 10:100
14. Ecker Y., Gilead M. (2018) Goal-Directed Allostasis: The Unique Challenge of Keeping Things as They Are and Strategies to Overcome It. Perspectives in Psychological Science 13(5) 618-633
15. Fogel A. (2000) Restorative Embodiment and Resilience: A Guideto Disrupr=t Habits, Create Inner Peace, Deepen Relationships, and Feel Greater Presence. North Atlantic Books, Berkeley, California.
16. Gibson J. (2019) Mindfullness, Interoception, and the Body: A Contemporary Perspective. Front. Psychol 10:2012
17. Halvorson H.G. (2012) 9 Things Successful People Do. Harvard Business Review Press, Boston, Mass.
18. Hargaden H. & Sills, C. (2002) Transactional Analysis: A Relational Perspective. New York: Routledge.
19. Kleckner I.R., et al, (2017) Evidence for a large-scale brain system supporting allostasis and interocpetion in humans. Nature Human Behaviour 1: 0069

# REFERENCES (cont.)

1. McParlin Z., Cerritelli F., Friston K.J., Esteves J.E. (2022) Therapeutic Alliance as Active Inference: The Role of Therapeutic Touch and Synchrony. Frontiers in Psychology, 10:3389.
2. Nagoski E. and Nagasaki A. (2019), Burnout: The Secret to Unlocking the Stress Cycle.Vermillon, London.
3. Ogden P. Fisher J.(2015) Sensorimotor Psychotherapy: Interventions for Trauma and Attachment. Norton, NY.
4. Pink D. (2009), Drive. Canongate, Edin.
5. Porges S. (2011) PolyVagal Theory. Norton, NY.
6. Porges S. (2009) Polyvagal theory: New insights inot adaptive reactions of the autonomic nervous system, Cleveland Clin. J. Med 76: (supple 2): S86-S90.
7. ter Kuile C.(2020) The Power Of Ritual. William Collins, London.
8. Treleaven, D.A. (2018) Trauma Sensitive Mindfulness. Norton, NY.
9. Schulkin J., Sterling P. (2019) Allostasis: A Brain-Centred, Predictive Model of Physiological Regulation. Trends in Neuroscience 42:10
10. Wang Z. (2021) The entropy perspective on human illness and aging. Engineering 08-014
11. Weng H.Y., et al (2021) Interventions and Manipulations of Interoception Trends in Neuroscience 44:1
12. Winfrey O. (2019), The Path Made Clear: Dus=iscovering Your Life's Direction nd Purpose. Bluebird Books For Life, Pan McMillan.

Effect of HIIT Workouts on Cortisol
ttps://journals.plos.org/plosone/article?id=10.1371/journal.pone.0243276
https://journals.lww.com/nsca-jscr/Fulltext/2013/03000/Adrenal_Cortical_Responses_to_High_Intensity

Grounding
REF: https://pubmed.ncbi.nlm.nih.gov/36528336/
https://pubmed.ncbi.nlm.nih.gov/22291721/
https://pubmed.ncbi.nlm.nih.gov/18047442/